PRACTISING HEALTH PROMOTION

Dilemmas and Challenges

Jennie Naidoo
Senior Lecturer, Health Promotion,
University of the West of England, Bristol, UK

and

Jane Wills
Senior Lecturer, Health Promotion,
South Bank University, London, UK

Baillière Tindall

PUBLISHED IN ASSOCIATION WITH THE RCN

London   Philadelphia   Toronto   Sydney   Tokyo

BAILLIÈRE TINDALL
An imprint of Harcourt Brace and Company Limited

© Harcourt Brace and Company Limited 1998

First published 1998
   Reprinted 1999

ISBN 07020 2122 9

British Library Cataloguing in Publication Data
A catalogue record for this book is available from the British Library

Library of Congress Cataloging in Publication Data
A catalog record for this book is available from the Library of Congress

Printed in China

The
Publisher's
policy is to use
**paper manufactured
from sustainable forests**
II

*C*ontents

Acknowledgements

Our first book *Health Promotion: Foundations for Practice* was published three years ago, so we knew what was involved in writing another book, but had forgotten the intensity of the experience. We would like to thank our families and friends who have supported us through this time yet again.

There are numerous colleagues and students whose ideas have informed this book. There are too many to mention but particular thanks are due to Judy Orme, Tricia Parsons, Laura Markowe, Oxford branch of Society of Health Promotion Specialists, Don Rawson, Mark Maguire, Jo Harris and Fiona Bower. We hope that this book represents the vigour of their debates and will continue to stimulate discussion and motivate health promotion practitioners.

In particular we would like to thank the practitioners who wrote or contributed material for the chapters in Part 3:

Jeremy Cole MSc, DipHEd
Health Promotion Adviser (Accident Prevention), East Sussex, Brighton and Hove Health Authority, Eastbourne

Deborah Loeb BA(Hons), MSc (Health Promotion)
Principal Health Promotion Adviser, Community Relations and Health Promotion, East London and the City Health Authority, London

Wolfgang Markham BSc(Hons), MPhil, PhD
Research Fellow, School of Education, University of Birmingham, Birmingham

Jo Mussen BA(Hons), PGCE, MSc (Health Promotion)
Formerly Senior Health Promotion Specialist, Health Promotion Service of Camden & Islington Community Health Services NHS Trust, London; Health Promotion Service Coordinator, Shropshire Community Health Services NHS Trust, Shrewsbury

Vicki Taylor BSc(Hons), MA, MSc, PGCE
Assistant Director, Health Promotion Commissioning and Health Strategy, Camden & Islington Health Authority, London

*P*reface

Health promotion is a relatively new field. In 1980, the year in which the Black Report on inequalities in health was published, there was relatively little academic writing on health promotion. Indeed, the term health education was most often used reflecting the belief that it was important to educate and persuade people to change their health behaviour. Since that time there has been a lively debate about the purpose and practice of health promotion although there is no consensus about what should be done to promote the nation's health. In the 1980s the World Health Organization (Health For All, 1985; Ottawa Charter, 1986) called for a wider approach to promoting health in which the circumstances and environments in which people live would be changed to create opportunities for people to choose healthier options. From a relatively narrow focus on changing people's behaviour, health promotion had become a broad and complex field encompassing policy change and community action. Promoting health is now, to some extent, everybody's business. It is not just a concern of the NHS but also of all those involved in health and welfare work, education and environmental protection. Many practitioners find such a broad approach daunting and find it difficult to identify how to include health promotion in their practice. This book aims to offer practitioners guidelines and examples of effective health promotion in order to progress their practice.

Since 1990 the NHS, in which much health promotion work takes place, has undergone radical change. England, Scotland, Wales and Ireland have national health strategies which include specific targets for reducing illness and disease and working for health gain. Primary care has been prioritized with the intention of channelling resources through this sector. There is an increasing emphasis in all health work on justifying its practice according to evidence of effectiveness. The Labour government, formed in May 1997, has committed itself to taking a broad view on how the nation's health can be improved. The national health strategy is to be revised so that it recognizes the significance of poverty and inequality in producing ill health. The challenge for practitioners is to reconcile the principles outlined by the World Health Organization – equity, community participation, intersectoral collaboration and the need to reorientate health away from solely medical care – with the narrow lifestyle focus in which health promotion is often viewed.

In our first book *Health Promotion: Foundations for Practice* we reviewed some of the knowledge and skills with which practitioners need to be familiar in order to promote health and looked at some examples of differing approaches to this task. In this book we explore further what should inform the practice of health promotion. We suggest that health promotion practice should be informed by theory and certain core principles and that practitioner know-how alone is an insufficient basis for health promotion. Schon (1983) has presented a powerful argument that practitioners need to become engaged in "reflection-in-action" as well as "knowing-in-action" if they are to improve and enhance their practice. Practitioners should undertake continual evaluation of their work through critical analysis and extend their theoretical understanding by reflection on applied experience. This book explores those principles, tenets and practices of health promotion which we feel from our experience of working in and teaching health promotion over many years, are problematic. Our aim is to enable health promoters from different backgrounds and within different settings to clarify the dilemmas and challenges which arise from attempting to put theory into practice and in so doing to advance their practice.

This book is organized into three parts. Part 1 explores the nature of health promotion as a discipline and the kinds of knowledge upon which health promotion is based. The three chapters consider how a reflective practitioner can integrate research and evidence of effectiveness into their work. Part 2 examines how the core principles for health promotion proposed by the World Health Organization can be incorporated into practice. The resulting dilemmas are identified and discussed. Part 3 takes five key issues which have been deemed national priorities because they constitute major causes of mortality and ill health. Practitioners from the field have co-authored these chapters offering their perspectives on the approaches that can be taken to promote health and reduce ill health in these areas.

The book is clearly structured and signposted for ease of reading and study. Each chapter starts with an overview outlining the contents of that chapter and its links with other chapters and a few key points. Interspersed throughout the text are a number of helpful features:

Example (**E**)
Case study (**C**)
Activity (**A**)
Reflection point (**R**)
Discussion point (**D**).

Jennie Naidoo
Jane Wills

References

Schon D (1983) *The reflective practitioner*, London, Temple Smith.

World Health Organization (1985) *Targets for Health for All*, Copenhagen, WHO Regional Office for Europe.

World Health Organization (1986) "The Ottawa charter for health promotion". *Health Promotion*, **1**, iii–v.

PART 1

Theory and Practice

Introduction

Chapter 1 examines the body of theory and some of the key principles which inform health promotion and why their application to practice is difficult. Chapter 2 discusses the evidence and research which informs health promotion. It shows how evidence linking ill-health to socio-economic conditions is often ignored. Rather, the reliance on epidemiology leads health promotion to focus on addressing risk factors for disease, and practitioners are called upon to justify their work by focusing on behavioural outcomes. Chapter 3 discusses the current emphasis on evidence-based practice and the criteria for effectiveness which are used to evaluate health promotion. It argues that the current trend of borrowing scientific criteria from medicine is not always appropriate for health promotion, and that there is a need to integrate methodology from the social sciences.

1 *Theory into practice*

Key points

- Health promotion and professional roles.
- Process and principles.
- Skills for health promotion and reflective practice.
- Defining health promotion theory.
- Theoretical tensions in health promotion.

Overview

An understanding of health promotion theory is essential to informed practice. Yet identifying the body of theory that informs health promotion is difficult and applying theory to practice is not straightforward. Many occupational groups claim a role in promoting health. Yet each may draw from a different knowledge base (biomedicine, education, psychology, social sciences) and have a different perspective on what constitutes health promotion. This chapter argues that practitioners should be aware of the underpinning knowledge base of health promotion and the values implicit in the approach they adopt. In so doing practitioners begin to clarify their view of the purpose of health promotion and which strategies are suggested by different aims. Otherwise practitioners merely respond to practice imperatives and their health promotion work is limited to narrow tasks.

Introduction

Health promotion is generally taken to be an umbrella term that includes all those activities intended to prevent disease, improve health and enhance well-being. Health and well-being are both contested concepts and health promoters may not have a shared understanding of what constitutes health. The dominant definition of health is as "the absence of disease". But for many practitioners health means mental, social and emotional health and well-being, as well as physical health.

Uncertainty surrounding the concept of health makes unpacking the concept of health promotion difficult. Some authors have attempted to define health promotion by tracing its historical development as a field of activity and its roots in public health policy and health education (e.g. Bunton and Macdonald, 1992). Other authors have taken a philosophical perspective and attempted to define health promotion by looking at the meanings of the terms health and promotion (e.g. Dines and Cribb, 1993). An alternative approach is to define the boundaries of practice (Ewles and Simnett, 1995).

Health, disease and illness, as well as being subjectively interpreted, are also influenced by a range of biological, psychological, environmental and social factors. This significantly affects the type of intervention developed to improve health. The intervention adopted will depend on the concept of health being used. For some practitioners the reduction or absence of disease is a principal aim; health promotion then centres around preventive medicine and influencing or persuading people to adopt healthier lifestyles. Others may see "health" more broadly as an aspect of fulfilled lives in which people achieve their potential. They may therefore seek to enable clients or groups to take more control over their lives. Others still may reject the notion of health as an individual responsibility and see "health" as a social value and a fundamental right. To promote health is to address the root causes of ill-health in the physical, social and economic environment and to work on the "building blocks" for health, such as housing, employment and nutrition.

Although health promotion is a clearly defined function within the NHS, there is a lack of consensus about its definition and how it is to be implemented. Health promotion may take place at the level of individuals, communities, policies and structures. It is possible to distinguish four elements in the "field" of health promotion, although these are not necessarily discrete:

- **Disease prevention** – activities focusing on individuals or groups defined as at risk from a particular disease or condition, e.g. screening.
- **Health education and health information** – activities aimed at enhancing health and preventing disease through learning, e.g. mass media campaigns; practitioner–client consultations.
- **Public health promotion** – activities which seek to promote health through social and environmental measures, policy development and the equitable distribution of resources, e.g. the development of local partnerships; improved access to services.
- **Community development** – activities which enable individuals to develop their personal skills, knowledge and social networks, and for communities to identify and link with service providers to meet their health needs, e.g. women's health groups; residents' groups; mental health user groups.

Health promotion and professional roles

Health promotion has become "everybody's business". Many practitioners now have "health promotion" identified as an aspect of their work. Yet just as there is no single account of what health promotion is, so there is no single discrete area of activity that is health promotion.

E xample

Professional roles and health promotion

Nurses, midwives and health visitors
". . . incorporate into their professional care, whether in hospital or community, activities related to the promotion of health, prevention of disease, and an approach which encourages individuals to take responsibility for their own health" (RCN, 1989).

General practitioners
The 1996 revised contract for health promotion allows GPs to set their own proposals for carrying out funded health promotion activities for their practice population. These proposals are agreed and monitored by local health promotion committees which include doctor representatives.

Teachers
". . . promote the spiritual, moral, cultural, mental and physical development of pupils" (Section 1 1988 Education Reform Act).

Environmental health officers
". . . have a special part to play with their responsibilities for health and safety at work, food safety and food quality and in collaboration with health authorities for health promotion and investigating and bringing under control outbreaks of communicable disease" (Department of Health, 1992).

R   Which other practitioners can you think of whose work is expected to promote health?

Most of these areas of practice regard themselves as professions in that they have specialized knowledge and training, and are self-regulating, i.e. only those assessed as competent are allowed to practise (Freidson, 1970). Health promotion is not a profession. Whilst there are qualifications in health promotion, specialist practitioners in the NHS (Health Education/Promotion Specialists or Advisers) and specialist health promotion services, the practice of health promotion is not exclusive to this group. Neither is there a licence to practise or mandatory registration for health promotion specialists. So, when practitioners claim to be health promoters, is there a shared understanding of goals and methods and on what do they base their practice?

Many professional groups have integrated health promotion into their practice. It has been claimed enthusiastically, particularly by nurses. A major review of the professional education and training of all branches of nursing (Project 2000) in the 1980s reflected a shift to a more holistic view of health. There was recognition of the need to move away from a single practitioner–single patient approach to one of greater partnership with clients and more work in and with communities (UKCC, 1986).

R How do you think your professional group interprets health promotion?

How practitioners interpret their health promotion role will depend on many factors including their professional training, their role in the organization, their personal experience, interests and social and political perspective. For some, health promotion is an *activity*. Public health and health promotion specialists have a strategic role in needs assessment and setting targets for health gain. They may also provide programmes of training, education and support to other professionals and the community. General practices may provide screening services and lifestyle advice. (Chapter 7 explores in detail how health promotion is interpreted in primary health care).

Gott and O'Brien (1990) in their study of nurses and health promotion found that all nurses, whether hospital based or in the community, emphasize lifestyle interventions in their work. Usually this is done through the transmission of information and it may also include screening for risk factors for specific disease conditions. Nurses regarded communication skills and the quality of the nurse–patient relationship as their most significant contribution to health promotion. Gott and O'Brien (1990) argue that the nursing process encourages nurses to identify individual problems and therefore the ability to understand health as an interrelationship between social and political factors as well as biomedical and psychological factors is rare:

> "'facilitate', 'enable' and 'empower' is being interpreted in practice as communicating to people what their risks of specific diseases are, then further communicating what people should do to reduce these" (Gott and O'Brien 1990:14).

For most practitioners, health promotion activities are additional to their primary role. Its inclusion in their remit poses an additional burden of work and extra time, resulting in it becoming "bolted on" rather than integral to their way of working.

Process and principles

R What do you see as your health promotion role? What activities do you carry out? What specific bodies of knowledge do you use in your everyday practice to guide and inform your actions?

Health promotion may not be identified as specific activities but more about a process which influences the way practitioners carry out their traditional role. To work in a health promoting way means:

- **A focus on health not illness** – working with the well not just the sick, enhancing well-being not merely reducing or alleviating illness.
- **Empowering clients** – enabling individuals and groups to have a say in how their health is to be promoted and recognizing the value of their perspective; supporting people to acquire the skills and confidence to take greater control of their own health.
- **Recognizing that health is multidimensional** – mental, social, emotional, spiritual and sexual needs are as important as

physical ones and the whole person and their needs must be taken into account.

■ **Acknowledging that health is influenced by factors outside individual control** – trying to address the root causes of ill-health and not "blaming the victim".

If health promotion is a process and it is possible to carry out work in a health promoting way, how would a practitioner know if they were doing this? One of the characteristics of a profession is that there is a code of conduct, the purpose of which is to persuade the public that the occupation can be trusted and acts with integrity. Codes of Conduct derive from the values which underpin that profession. The Codes of Professional Conduct for most health and welfare practitioners include as a central tenet a respect for autonomy. Other principles which follow from this include individual liberty and choice, empowerment of individuals or groups, and public participation in decisions which affect health.

Activity

> The World Health Organization outlined a set of guiding principles with which to orientate health promotion work as part of its commitment to Health for All by the Year 2000 (WHO, 1985):
>
> 1. Equity.
> 2. Empowerment.
> 3. Community participation.
> 4. Multisectoral collaboration.
> 5. Emphasis on primary healthcare.
>
> ■ What kind of tasks or services would be developed by adherence to these principles?
> ■ Are these appropriate goals for your work?
> ■ What other principles or values guide your work?
> ■ Are the principles you came up with distinctive and specific to health work or are they more general notions such as "respect" or "enhancing quality of life"?

In Part Two we look at how some of these principles are incorporated into practice. Chapter 4 discusses the concept of equity and the implications for resource allocation and service provision which is based on need. Chapter 7 examines how patients can be involved in decision making in general practice and discusses the concept of participation. Chapter 8 explores the local partnerships between statutory agencies and voluntary and community groups and discusses the opportunities for collaboration provided by the need to look at future sustainable development.

Skills for health promotion and reflective practice

As we have seen, an increasing range of practitioners see themselves as promoting health. What then are the skills that are necessary for health promotion? There will be practitioners who believe that health promotion, like many other occupations in health and social care, is essentially about practice and "knowing how to". Anti-intellectualism is prevalent in many occupations, with practitioners valuing their client relationship and "good old-fashioned caring" above macro level social change. Where an occupation is relatively diffuse, as in health promotion, practitioners often try to characterize the activity in terms of its competencies.

D What do health promoters need to be able to do?

Although the specific role of health promoters will vary according to their position within the NHS purchaser/provider structure, the skills necessary for carrying out this work can be broadly outlined:

■ **Research** – identifying needs and priorities, evaluating the value and cost-effectiveness of interventions, using market research to target information.
■ **Communication** – interpersonal skills, writing, working with the media.
■ **Organization and management** – management of time, people and resources, working in teams, networking and liaison, setting up and supporting health alliances and partnerships, managing change, commissioning health promotion, planning and project management.
■ **Education and training** – supporting and leading groups, teaching and facilitating.
■ **Publicity and media** – developing or providing appropriate resources and material, raising public awareness through campaigns.

R ■ Do any of these skills for health promotion surprise you?
■ Are there any you would add?

As health promotion becomes more prominent in practitioners' roles, it is necessary to identify the key skills for health promotion work. What is surprising is that many of these skills are generic ones and apply to all health and welfare work, e.g. communication, planning, networking. The Occupational Standards Council for Health and Social Care (the Care Sector Consortium) is currently developing standards of competence for the health and social care field and these will include occupational standards for health promotion. Competency-based programmes as a measure of quality have been the basis for the establishment of the National Council for Vocational Qualifications (NCVQs). The impetus has come from the development of craft and technical education based on the need for a skilled workforce. It was therefore thought necessary that people should be able to demonstrate their ability to carry out certain tasks and that they had transferable skills.

The concept of competence has severe limitations, however, when applied to an occupation such as health promotion. One of the main difficulties is specifying the competencies involved. Competencies cannot cover all types of activities nor the personal processes entailed in the practice of health promotion. To be a health promoter is not merely to possess a set of skills but to implement them in a health promoting way and this is very hard to demonstrate. In specifying a range of activities in which the practitioner must perform, the role of theory and understanding is diminished. "Knowing" becomes merely preparation for "doing" with no requirement to reflect on theoretical bases or make sense of working practice.

Does it matter if practitioners don't have a theoretical base for what they do? In one sense it doesn't – theoretical understanding is not a recipe for success and it cannot provide answers to what practitioners should do. The explicit use of theory by practitioners is not common despite Kurt Lewin's oft quoted statement that "There is nothing as practical as a good theory". The reality is that for most practitioners theory is unrealistic and inapplicable in the face of the stark realities of day-to-day practice. Many practitioners adopt a pragmatic or common sense approach.

D

> What is the common sense that underpins health promotion?
> "People just need to know what's good for them";
> "Practitioners just need to find the best ways of telling people";
> "Middle class people are more educated and understand how to look after themselves";
> "We need to understand peoples attitudes so we can change them".

But as Thompson points out:

> " . . . common sense is ideological – it serves to reinforce traditional values and the inequalities associated with these. It is based on implicit assumptions and if we rely on common sense to guide our thoughts, we are not in a position to question those assumptions" (Thompson, 1995:28).

R What traditional values and associated inequalities do you think are exemplified in the above quotations?

It is often assumed that there is **a** healthy way of living and practitioners focus on the individual or individuals with the aim of changing their behaviour to this end. Research on health status has shown however, that the "healthier choice" is not available to all (e.g. Benzeval *et al.*, 1995). Thus people may be blamed for health behaviours over which they do not have control. The simple equation that knowledge + attitudes = behaviour has also formed the basis of much health education work, yet the provision of information alone is unlikely to change behaviour. The giving of information can re-inforce the expert status of the practitioner and fail to provide for the active participation of clients in an education process which addresses issues of concern to them. Middle class, educated people are often seen as "easier" clients and so are targeted more (yet need it least). When practitioners do not derive their practice from a theoretical framework, the practice wisdom regarded as "common sense" tends to reinforce simplistic assumptions which serve to re-inforce inequalities.

Theory is perceived by many practitioners to be book learning. Many practitioners value received wisdom – "we do it like this" – and learning on the job over an intellectual understanding of the practice process. To know "how to" is more important than to "know why". This issue has been vehemently debated in recent years by those involved in professional education. Nurse educators have expressed concern that less time is spent on the wards and more emphasis is being placed on research-based knowledge. Those involved in teacher education have expressed equal concern about the reverse situation – that more time is to be spent in classrooms and less on the theoretical underpinning of education!

Activity

> Consider the following opposing viewpoints on the importance of theory in health promotion. Which comes closest to your own view? What further arguments could you use to support this view? (You might want to debate this with a colleague.)
>
> A. Theory isn't important in health promotion. Accounts of inter-ventions show little evidence of them having been based on theory. Doing health promotion is just common sense and experience. The skills gained in previous training are quite adequate for our health promotion role. We just need to find out the best way of getting through to people. All this high flown stuff is unrealistic.
> B. It's important that our work does derive from a sound know-ledge-base. We need to be able to see why we do it the way we do and to be able to explain this to others who may have a different view. Understanding theory helps to clarify the purpose and effec-tiveness of health promotion and makes it less likely to suffer contradictions.

In such a complex and evolving field as health promotion an under-standing of theory assumes great importance:

- It gives a common method and language through which to con-duct a more thorough and informed debate (Caplan, 1993:156).
- It gives credibility to practice and gives the practitioner the con-fidence to justify their choice of action when confronted with dif-fering interpretations of health promotion by colleagues, managers or politicians.

- It gives health promotion practice a professional identity.
- It provides explanations which are based on empirical reality and a tool for more logical and coherent practice.

The professional education of many practitioners, particularly in health and education, has been dominated in recent years by the work of Schon and the concept of the "reflective practitioner". Schon (1983) characterizes professional practice as the high ground of research and theory and a swampy lowland that is the messy, confusing problems of everyday practice. He likens many practitioners to the jazz musician or cook who is highly skilled at what they do and because of their experience is able to improvise but who may not know or understand the theoretical basis of musical syncopation or the emulsification of fats. Schon argues that through reflection-in-action a practitioner learns the tricks of the trade and what works in practice. Schon also says however, that practitioners need to be able to reflect **on** action and to remove themselves from the swamp of practice and take a broad view. The reflective practitioner is able to integrate these two aspects. The reflective practitioner uses theory, understanding how it may help in their practice and how their experience can become part of a wider theoretical understanding.

> "Those responsible for health promotion should be able to describe the philosophical aspects of what they are trying to do, and some guiding principles, as well as the values and ethics involved." (Evans *et al.*, 1994:10)

 Activity

Think of a health promotion action which you have taken recently, or a health promotion programme that you have been part of, about which you felt uncertain or confused. Figure 1.1 shows a cycle of questions to encourage you to reflect on this experience and identify any learning points from it and how other learning can help you to make sense of it.

Through this process, links are made between experience and theory and practice. Kolb (1984) argued that if we are to learn effectively, experience needs to be carefully and systematically reflected upon. Practitioners and students in classroom situations who focus on an "experience" or a situation about which they felt uncomfortable may begin to understand the ways in which their knowledge was inadequate for the situation. Through sharing that information they can discover how others experience in a different way something they may have taken for granted. Through analysing or interpreting the issue or situation they can abstract general principles from it. By drawing on theoretical frameworks they can see what further knowledge may be required, and then apply this back to their practice, perhaps trying out new ideas or doing things a different way. The whole process is a cycle of practice–theory–practice or PRAXIS.

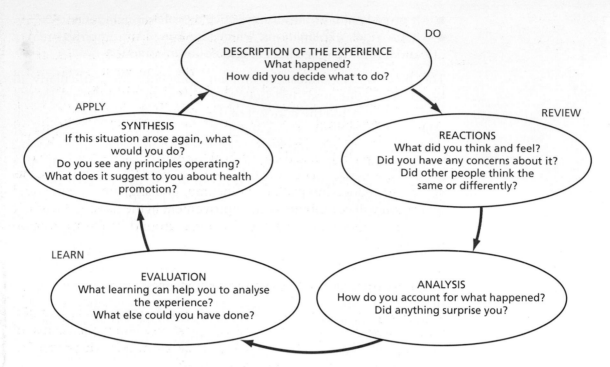

Figure 1.1 *The Cycle of Reflection.*

Schon (1983) argues that "technical rationality" dominates professional thinking. But it is important that practitioners think about *why* things are done in the way they are, *how* they could be done differently and *what* they are trying to achieve. Practitioners may believe they can apply their professional knowledge to select the best method for their purposes. But the problems of the real world (and the practice of health promotion is no exception) do not present as neatly parcelled issues. When practitioners decide the form of their health promotion activity they are also choosing to frame the issue in a particular way which may mean reconciling, integrating or choosing among different interpretations and approaches. The action they take reflects particular aims and values – particular beliefs about health, about the influences on people's health and about the role of the practitioner.

D

Consider the following question: Which are the three main issues facing health promotion in the 1990s?
Was your answer framed in terms of:

■ diseases and conditions, e.g. AIDS, heart disease, asthma
■ lifestyles, e.g. smoking, unhealthy eating, drug use
■ wider social issues, e.g. poverty, housing and homelessness, pollution
■ professional practice issues, e.g. effectiveness, evaluation, funding.

How you frame your answer to the above Discussion point reflects what forms of knowledge are most dominant for you. There are obviously no right or wrong answers to this, but it is crucial for health promoters to consider who is deciding what constitutes a health promotion issue and what theoretical knowledge is being used to frame the issues. It is likely that most practitioners work within a biomedical paradigm and framed their answers to this in terms of diseases or risk factors. The dominant health promotion discourse in the UK is based on medical knowledge and centres on risk factors for diseases. The new Labour government has claimed that its actions to reduce inequalities in income, housing, employment and education will contribute to an improvement in the nation's health. It is possible, therefore, that the discourse around health promotion may change.

Understanding health promotion theory

The attempt to conceptualize health promotion beyond a set of activities, competencies or skills raises questions about the status of health promotion as a field of study. What knowledge do practitioners draw on to practise health promotion?

D

> Mr Jones is 76 and has leg ulcers. He is in the early stages of Alzheimer's Disease and lives alone since the death of his wife in the previous year. The District Nurse visits Mr Jones daily to dress his leg and draws upon her technical knowledge to do so, regarding herself as a competent practitioner. She is aware that she must include Mr Jones' health needs in her nursing assessment.
>
> - How does the District Nurse begin?
> - What factors will influence how she "frames" the health promotion aspects of her work?

The District Nurse might regard health promotion as integral to her care of Mr Jones or she might regard it as an additional task to be "bolted on" to her essential work. She might see her role as enabling Mr Jones to keep himself safe and in good health, or as preventing harm or disease from befalling him. Whichever role she prioritizes will affect her activities. If her priority is safety and good health she might advise Mr Jones about a healthy diet and safety precautions and spend considerable time talking to Mr Jones in order to enhance his capacities. She might enlist the services of voluntary and self-help organizations and try to broaden Mr Jones' social contacts. If her priority is to prevent disease or harm, she might focus on providing support for Mr Jones in the form of Meals on Wheels and cooking and bathing aids.

This example illustrates how practitioners work in different paradigms. A paradigm can be defined as "a way of knowing" and thereby interpreting a field of study characterized by particular beliefs and values, by particular theories and ways of problem solving and by particular methods and tools that are used in practice. The paradigm within which many health promoters work is that of Western science which has a mechanistic view of the body and views health as the antithesis of disease. Within this paradigm there are several theories or sets of propositions that explain or predict events such as theories about behaviour change or risk factors for disease. Health promoters may work in different paradigms, drawing upon different theories, and this will depend on their role, their professional background and training and their personal beliefs and interests.

C ase study

Using theory to inform practice

An occupational health nurse set up a workplace health and activity programme. Based on her common sense belief that everyone wants to protect their health, the programme combined an educational input stressing the risks to health from lack of exercise and excessive weight. Opportunities for change were provided through a programme of exercises, monitoring of exercise recovery rates, and food diaries. She also persuaded the company to pay employees half time rates for attending the programme. The programme was quite successful but many employees did not participate, some dropped out and few managed to maintain an activity programme for themselves.

When planning a subsequent programme, the occupational health nurse drew particularly on social cognitive theory and the concept of value expectancy which states that people are likely to take some action if they believe the action will be effective and if they value the action's results (Ajzen, 1988). The occupational health nurse thus realized that a vague promise of better health in the future didn't mean as much to the employees as it did to her in her professional role. Through informal discussions she learned that the participants' values related to "feeling more attractive", "wearing different clothes", "being able to take part in sports and exercise". Social cognitive theory also helped her to understand the importance of boosting participants' confidence in their ability to take up and maintain an exercise programme. This resulted in her introducing smaller targeted group sessions which combined exercise and discussion of health related topics (adapted from Hochbaum, 1992).

In the example above, the practitioner drew on theories from social psychology and used them as a tool to help her question her purpose and consider the most appropriate methods for her programme. There are various sets of explanations practitioners draw on to help them decide how to promote health:

- How people learn.
- How people make decisions and change their behaviour.
- How society is organized and how social structures influence health.
- How messages are communicated and can be targeted to particular groups.

These theories derive from many different disciplines. Rawson (1992) has described health promotion as a "borrowed discipline" importing theories from other bodies of knowledge such as sociology and psychology. This gives health promotion the appearance of a mish-mash of ideas, lacking credibility. But there is a powerful case being made in professional journals, in academic courses and in the field to suggest that although health promotion draws from other disciplines, applying these disciplines to its own field creates a discrete body of knowledge with its own theoretical base. Bunton and Macdonald (1992) suggest that health promotion is a multidisciplinary endeavour and that different forms of knowledge add to health promotion, consolidating it into a distinct discipline. Rawson (1992) in the same volume has argued that the diversity of health promotion reflects the contested nature of the concepts of health and education and its brief history as an occupation.

Activity

Health promotion – a borrowed discipline?
(Source: Bunton and Macdonald, 1992)

- Consider the ways in which the disciplines outlined below contribute to health promotion.
- To what extent is the eclectic nature of health promotion a strength? What are the drawbacks?

Psychology
Social learning theory, attribution theory and the health belief model help us to understand and explain human behaviour essential to health and the ways in which individuals make health-related decisions about, for example, taking up exercise, using a condom or changing drinking patterns. Psychological theories of mass communication in the 1960s, which assumed a direct link between knowledge, attitudes and behaviour, are still widely adhered to despite the ineffectiveness of programmes based on this premise.

Sociology
In analysing how society is organized and the social processes within it, we can examine the social role of medicine and how health and illness have come to be defined. An analysis of power and control and an understanding of the relationship between social structures and individual action helps us to consider how changes to promote health might come about. An analysis of the way in which society is stratified helps health promoters to consider how individual behaviour is constrained and influenced.

Education

Philosophers argue that the fundamental aim of education is to increase autonomy and to initiate learners into "ways of knowing". Freedom to choose and the acceptance of other peoples' ways of knowing are fundamental to the practice of health promotion. Psychology has also shaped health promotion practice in helping us to understand how people learn and how to develop strategies to involve people in their own learning. Educational theory is used to plan and evaluate those processes intended to have a learning outcome, usually a change in knowledge, attitude or skills.

Public health medicine

Epidemiology contributes understanding about the aetiology of disease and the effectiveness of preventive medicine. Epidemiology is based on a medical science model, although increasingly there have been calls to establish a "social epidemiology of health" (Badura and Kickbusch, 1991). The study of risk factors for disease and health should, it is argued, go beyond traditional lifestyle or medical factors, to embrace factors such as degree of social networks and isolation and socially-produced stress.

Models of health promotion

One way of conceptualizing health promotion and integrating different disciplines is by using models. During the 1980s the attempts to define and clarify the practice of health promotion generated a vigorous debate in which academics and practitioners attempted to represent the sets of ideas which contributed to health promotion. In 1988 Rawson identified about 20 different models of health promotion (Rawson and Grigg, 1988).

A model is a way of bridging the gap between theory and practice. It helps practitioners to stand back and make sense of the complexity and reality of practice by mapping the strategic choices they face. Models of health promotion derive from different theories about health, education, individual and social change and the relationship between them. As the field changes and definitions of health promotion shift, so new models emerge which attempt to incorporate these new perspectives.

Different models of health promotion may:

■ conceptualize or map the field of health promotion;
■ interrogate and analyse existing practice;
■ plan and chart the possibilities for interventions.

Ewles and Simnett's (1995) model is widely used by practitioners planning a programme to address a particular issue. It describes five approaches to health promotion based on their observations of practice. It is a neutral model which makes no judgement about the relative worth of any of these approaches. Other models such as that of Beattie (1993) are taxonomies of different approaches and can be used to analyse practice or as a tool to look at the dilemmas of choice and how different social and political values give rise to different interventions.

Beattie describes the model as useful in "charting and selecting the particular mix of approaches that make up a programme or project and also in exploring and reviewing the ethical and political tensions within an intervention in terms of the balance of social values it encompasses" (Beattie, 1996:140). Beattie's model shows clearly how health promotion is embedded in the socio-cultural and political framework. It is not a technical activity in which practitioners merely choose the best strategy for improved health. The field of health promotion clearly reflects the tension between different value positions about power, knowledge, responsibility and autonomy. Beattie's model suggests there are four approaches for health promotion – (i) health persuasion, (ii) personal counselling for health, (iii) legislative action and (iv) community development. These paradigms arise from the relationship between the mode of intervention used (authoritative top-down or negotiated bottom-up) and the focus of the intervention (whether to individuals or communities).

Case study

Using Beattie's model

In this example, Beattie's model is used to show how it can help a practitioner to articulate her goals and to identify the particular methodologies that these goals entail. Beattie's model illustrates how different health promotion strategies are embedded in a distinctive paradigm for the professional–client relationship.

A midwife is considering how her practice can become more client-centred in the light of recommendations made by the Changing Childbirth report (DoH, 1993). She focuses on parent education classes which have been taking place in a similar form for some years. The midwife notes that the main aim of the parent classes is to "provide for the development of skilled, confident and informed parents"(Coombes and Schonveld, 1992). However, using Beattie's analysis she begins to question the parents' degree of control (Figure 1.2).

She notes that the content of classes is not negotiated with the women clients. Because those attending come from antenatal outpatients, there is no opportunity to establish a group and little attempt to identify needs. The midwife aims for the women to have successful deliveries – pregnancies brought to term; babies fit for discharge six hours after birth; good birth weights – medically determined outcomes which may not correspond to how a mother might define a satisfying and successful labour and birth. The midwife regards herself as

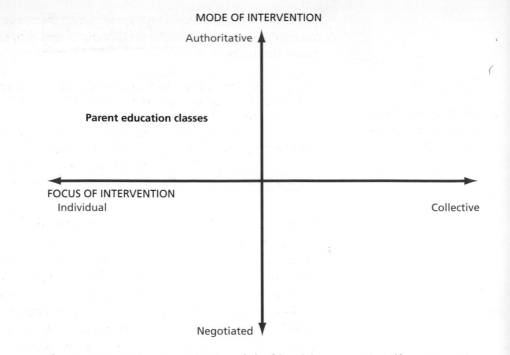

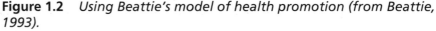

Figure 1.2   *Using Beattie's model of health promotion (from Beattie, 1993).*

empowering women. In her view, empowerment means giving women the information and resources to have a satisfying birth – what Beattie terms "The Prescriber". She sees how the biopathological model she adopted during her training and subsequent experience has encouraged her to see women as "at risk" or "in need". Her role is to remedy any "deficits" by providing information. The midwife acknowledges that she "frames" the issue as a medical one and that her years of experience lead her to see herself as the "expert" who can help mothers.

Although parent education classes are offered in groups and the midwife had been encouraged to shift her focus from individual client care to group work, the focus of attention is on the individual mother and not on women (or men) collectively as parents. The midwife recognizes that social factors such as low income and poor housing affect the health of mothers and children. However, the midwife's response is to regard these aspects as unchangeable apart from their effect on mothers' ability and willingness to change their lifestyles (e.g. smoking and diet). The mother is not seen as a whole person with a range of needs but as a pregnant woman to be "told" or "helped".

The hallmark of a reflective practitioner is to question accepted practice. Beattie's model is useful in helping the practitioner to identify the values and assumptions underlying her practice. It doesn't tell her what to do but it can help her to see what other possibilities there might be.

Activity

What alternative strategies can you suggest?

Figure 1.3 shows how Beattie's model can be used to generate possibilities for parent education and to explore how a practitioner might wish to shift her practice.

The model can also be used to generate the possible strategies there might be around an issue. Use Beattie's model to map the range of strategies regarding pregnant women who smoke. How could you use the model to argue your favoured approach?

So what is health promotion theory? Theories are products of their historical time and thus reflect a particular view of society. In health promotion, the dominance of theories about behaviour reflects the view that individuals are responsible for their own health. Such theories have provided the base for health promotion practice which seeks to influence and persuade people to change their attitudes and beliefs about their lifestyle. Gradually a critique of traditional health education has emerged and theories embedded in the concepts and principles of the WHO Health For All (1985) and Ottawa Charter

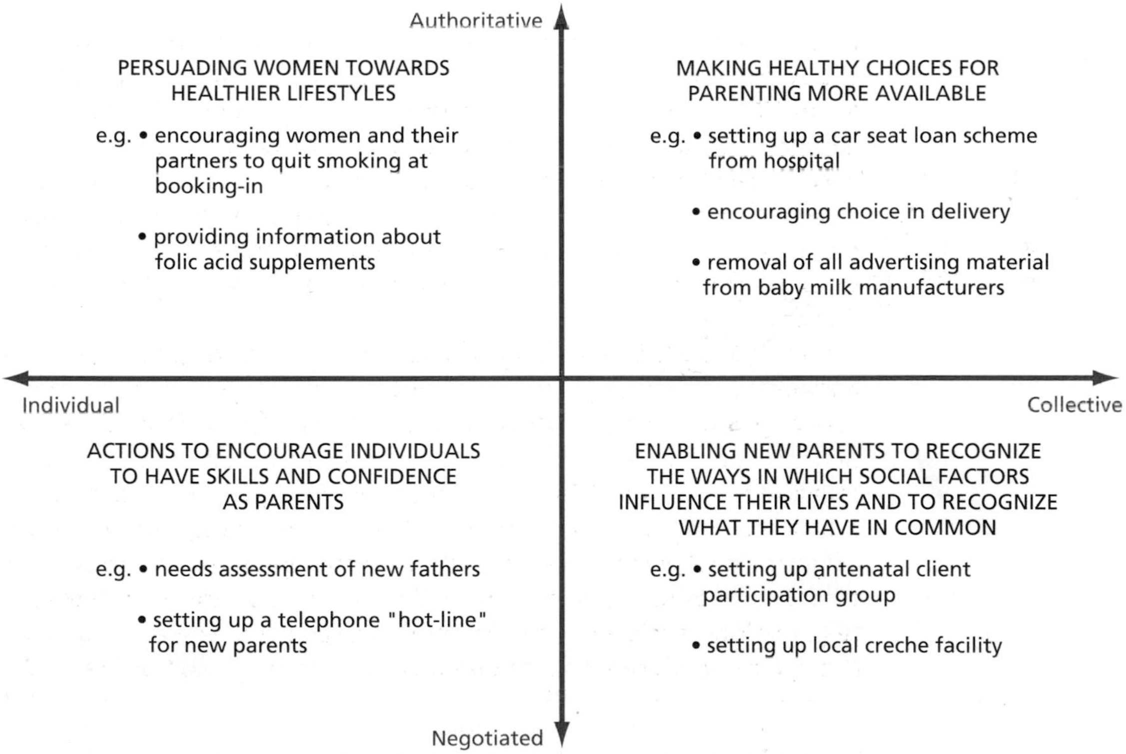

Authoritative

PERSUADING WOMEN TOWARDS
HEALTHIER LIFESTYLES

e.g. • encouraging women and their
partners to quit smoking at
booking-in

• providing information about
folic acid supplements

MAKING HEALTHY CHOICES FOR
PARENTING MORE AVAILABLE

e.g. • setting up a car seat loan scheme
from hospital

• encouraging choice in delivery

• removal of all advertising material
from baby milk manufacturers

Individual   Collective

ACTIONS TO ENCOURAGE INDIVIDUALS
TO HAVE SKILLS AND CONFIDENCE
AS PARENTS

e.g. • needs assessment of new fathers

• setting up a telephone "hot-line"
for new parents

ENABLING NEW PARENTS TO RECOGNIZE
THE WAYS IN WHICH SOCIAL FACTORS
INFLUENCE THEIR LIVES AND TO RECOGNIZE
WHAT THEY HAVE IN COMMON

e.g. • setting up antenatal client
participation group

• setting up local creche facility

Negotiated

Figure 1.3 *Generating alternative strategies; example of patient education.*

(WHO, 1986) were developed which place an emphasis on "environments, communities and policy and which encompassed the multi-level influences about the causal processes that people are exposed to in the context of daily living" (Dean, 1996)

D

What do you think is the basis of the critique of lifestyle health promotion?
And what is the critique of health promotion which seeks to promote Health For All?

Behavioural approaches to health promotion have received criticism because they are seen as victim-blaming, concerned with disease and for the most part, expert-led. Healthy lifestyles are seen as a simple matter of enabling an informed choice, taking little account of the social, physical and economic environment in which people live. The health promotion and Health For All movement has been criticized as social engineering. In going beyond simple information-giving and advice to addressing the structural causes of ill-health, health promotion begins to extend into all areas of people's lives. Targeting particular groups can be seen as trying to manipulate people's social norms and beliefs. As Kelly and Charlton (1995) put it, the paternalistic authority of the medical profession has given way to health promotion which has become the authority on the social causes of disease. Both the behavioural and the social perspective have been criticized as deterministic, suggesting that there is **a** cause for disease and ill-health.

Dissatisfaction with both of these traditional (or modern) accounts reached a peak in the 1980s and led to a new theoretical framework – post-modernism. Post-modernism questions whether any one explanatory model or overarching theory can explain health in society. The supremacy of science and medicine has been challenged. No longer is medicine seen as a wholly good thing which works to heal and restore – the damage to health through the side-effects of drug treatments and the loss of control engendered by dependency on doctors has led to widespread disillusion, reflected, in part, by the increased use of complementary therapies. Medicine's failure to halt or reduce many of the major causes of mortality reflects the limits of its capacity to cure. The social model based on theories of social divisions such as class, gender or ethnicity is seen as limited and insufficient, failing to account for many social inequalities or the complex interaction between them. A simple link between class and health is inadequate to explain why not all working class people get sick nor does it account for how people themselves explain their ill-health.

Example

The post-modernist approach

- Health is a contested concept which is the subject of many different and competing discourses, e.g. medical, popular, moral, legal, marketing. Each of these discourses constructs health in a particular way, which is relevant in different contexts and situations. Neither medicine nor a social model of health is sufficiently explanatory to account for the meaning of health in different contexts.
- Health is a relative concept which cannot be objectively defined as medicine has attempted to define disease. Expert discourses cannot explain why a person describes and makes sense of their experience of health and ill-health in the way they do. People's subjective meanings need to be valued.
- "The absence of disease" is inadequate as a definition of well-being. The person is a unique human subject with conscious and unconscious creative, sensual, aesthetic, spiritual, emotional selves. Working towards health needs to acknowledge the inter-relationship of all these dimensions of health.
- A person's health status or health experience cannot be "read off" their objective characteristics (such as gender or social class). Each situation and person is unique.

A post-modernist approach which rejects both structuralist and individualist frameworks of explanations for health and health status, but without offering any pointers for practice, may leave the practitioner at sea. If health isn't about the absence of disease (and health promotion therefore about working to prevent it) or about the inequalities produced by disadvantaged circumstances, then what is it? Using a broad approach which acknowledges each person's unique definition may lead to diversity but this is not necessarily an asset. It may lead to practitioners doing whatever is easiest which is usually reinforcing the status quo and more dominant forms of knowledge. It may also lead to relativism, where everything is seen as of equal value. In this book we will argue that this should not be the case for health promotion. Whilst structuralism can be critiqued and society has indeed become more complex, there are obvious and measurable differences and inequalities between social groups. A structural analysis does offer a useful framework for health promotion practice as it points up such differences for attention.

Conclusion

It is difficult to draw boundaries around health promotion and agree who is promoting health and what sorts of activities this entails. The attempt to mark out areas for specialists or to suggest that only qualified practitioners should practise health promotion reflects the need for health promotion, which is widely advocated but under-funded, to establish itself as a distinctive occupation and achieve the status and credibility accorded to a profession. Perhaps the most important aspect is to reflect on what we are doing in the name of health promotion and what it is we are trying to promote. Many authors despair of this debate:

> "There is a danger that obsessive concern with the meaning of 'health' can paralyse our activity and create sectarian divides between workers who should be cooperating. There will always be a wide range of activities that everyone agrees to be health promoting. We should get on with these tasks without waiting for agreement on all matters" (Kemm and Close, 1995:23).

As you will see in Part Two, it isn't as simple as just getting on with it. Influencing personal behaviour in a client encounter or a mass media campaign which seeks to shock may indeed be called health promotion but not everyone would agree that such activities are health promoting. Differing roles, professional backgrounds and funding constraints as much as ideology will influence the way in which a health promoter defines the purpose of health promotion. Our position is that health promotion needs to be based on sound theoretical underpinnings and adhere to certain core principles. In the rest of this book we explore how these principles might be put into practice and the sorts of dilemmas this throws up. It is from these dilemmas and trying to apply theory to practice that practitioners can learn and contribute to a developing field.

Further discussion

- A reflective practitioner is one who is capable of improving practice by "asking difficult questions and being sceptical of practices taken for granted" (Fitzgerald, 1994:75). In what ways are you incorporating reflective practice into your work?
- Consider a health promotion intervention with which you have been involved. What theoretical assumptions underpinned this activity? How would it be influenced by a consideration of other theoretical perspectives?

Recommended reading

- Bunton R and Macdonald G (1992) *Health promotion: Disciplines and Diversity*, London, Routledge.
  An important book which traces the theoretical roots of health promotion in disciplines such as psychology, sociology, education and epidemiology.

■ Bunton R, Nettleton S and Burrows R (eds) (1995) *Sociology of health promotion*, London, Routledge.
A stimulating book which takes a sociological perspective to health promotion with an interesting analysis of practice. The book includes some chapters on the implications of post-modernism for health promotion.

■ Gott M and O'Brien M (1990) *The Role of the Nurse in Health Promotion: Policies, Perspectives and Practice*, Buckingham, Open University Press.
A comprehensive research study funded by the Department of Health which examines the role of nurses in health promotion and their response to their expanded role.

■ Schon DA (1983) *The Reflective Practitioner*, London, Temple Smith.
The most important work to consider the process of reflection for learning in practice settings.

■ Additional literature on reflective practice in education, nursing and social welfare includes:
—Carr W and Kemmis S (1986) *Becoming critical: education, knowledge and action research,* London, Falmer Press.
—Gray G and Pratt R (1991) *Towards a discipline of nursing,* Melbourne, Churchill Livingstone.
—Palmer A, Burns S and Bulman C (eds) (1994) *Reflective Practice in Nursing,* Oxford, Blackwell Scientific.
—Thompson N (1995) *Theory and Practice in Health and Social Welfare,* Buckingham, Open University Press.
—Seedhouse D (1997) *Health Promotion: Philosophy, Prejudice and Practice*, Wiley, Chichester.
A fascinating and incisive, but personal, view of the conceptual roots of health promotion. The book argues that health promotion can only become a mature discipline when its purposes and philosophy are made clear.
—*Health Promotion International* (1996) (11)1.
Papers from a WHO workshop on theory in health promotion which explore the role of theory in health promotion and testing theory through lay perceptions.

References

Ajzen I (1988) *Attitudes, Personality and Behaviour*, Buckingham, Open University Press.

Badura B and Kickbusch I (1991) *Health Promotion Research: towards a new social epidemiology*, Geneva, WHO Regional Publications.

Beattie A (1993) "The changing boundaries of health", in Beattie A, Gott M, Jones L and Sidell M (eds) *Health and Wellbeing*, Basingstoke, Macmillan

Beattie A (1996) "The health promoting school: from idea to action", in Scriven A and Orme J (eds) *Health Promotion: Professional Perspectives,* Basingstoke, Macmillan.

Benzeval M, Judge K and Whitehead M (eds) (1995) *Tackling inequalities in health: an agenda for action,* London, Kings Fund.

Bunton R and Macdonald G (eds) (1992) *Health promotion: Disciplines and Diversity,* London, Routledge.

Caplan R (1993) "The importance of social theory for health promotion: from description to reflexivity", *Health Promotion International,* **8**(2), 147–57.

Coombes G and Schonveld (1992) *Life will never be the same again: a review of antenatal and postnatal health education,* London, Health Education Authority.

Dean K (1996) "Using theory to guide policy relevant to health promotion research", *Health Promotion International,* **11**(1), 19–26.

Department of Health (1992) *The Health of the Nation,* London, HMSO.

Department of Health (1993) *Changing childbirth: a survey of good communications practice in maternity services,* London, HMSO.

Dines A and Cribb A (1993) *Health Promotion: concepts and practice,* Oxford, Blackwell.

Evans D, Head MJ and Speller V (1994) *Good practice in health promotion: assuring quality in health promotion,* London, Health Education Authority.

Ewles L and Simnett I (1995) *Promoting Health: a practical guide,* London, Scutari.

Fitzgerald M (1994) "Theories of reflection for learning", in Palmer A (ed.) *Reflective Practice in Nursing,* Oxford, Blackwell.

Freidson E (1970) *The profession of medicine: a study of applied knowledge,* New York, Harper & Row.

Gott M and O'Brien M (1990) *The role of the nurse in health promotion: policies, perspectives and practice,* Buckingham, Department of Health/Open University.

Hochbaum GM (1992) "The role and uses of theory in health education practice", *Health Education Quarterly,* **19**(3).

Kelly M and Charlton B (1995) "The modern and the postmodern in health promotion", in Bunton R, Nettleton S and Burrows R (eds), *The sociology of health promotion: critical analyses of consumption, lifestyle and risk,* London, Routledge.

Kemm J and Close A (1995) *Health Promotion: Theory and Practice,* Basingstoke, Macmillan.

Kolb DA (1984) *Experiential learning – experience as the source of learning and development,* New Jersey, Prentice Hall.

Rawson D (1992) "The growth of health promotion theory and its rational reconstruction: lessons from the philosophy of science", in Bunton R and Macdonald G (eds), *Health promotion: Disciplines and Diversity,* London, Routledge.

Rawson D and Grigg C (1988) *Purpose and Practice in Health Education,* London, South Bank Polytechnic/Health Education Authority.

RCN (1989) *Into the 90s, promoting professional excellence,* London, Royal College of Nursing.

Schon D (1983) *The reflective practitioner,* London, Temple Smith.

Thompson N (1995) *Theory and Practice in Health and Social Welfare,* Buckingham, Open University Press.

UKCC (1986) *Project 2000: A New Preparation for Practice,* United Kingdom Central Council for Nursing, Midwifery and Health Visiting, London.

WHO (1985) *Targets for Health For All,* Copenhagen, World Health Organization.

WHO (1986) *Ottawa Charter for Health Promotion,* Ottawa, World Health Organization.

2 *Research for health promotion*

Key points

- Nature of research.
- Positivist and interpretive paradigms.
- Research for health promotion:
  - □ lay knowledge;
  - □ participative research;
  - □ social research.
- The researcher-practitioner.

Overview

Research is a link between theory and practice. It should, and does, inform practice but using such knowledge and applying it can be difficult. The greater emphasis on accountability in the NHS has led to calls for practice to become more evidence-based and, therefore, for practitioners to develop skills in research. This chapter looks at the nature of the research that informs health promotion. It argues that research for health promotion should provide the tools for tackling the social causes of ill-health and disease. This suggests the need for research methods that are participative, involving researchers and researched working together, and which explore lay people's knowledge and understanding of their own health. The chapter concludes by looking at the ways in which practitioners can become researchers themselves as well as active and critical consumers of research.

Introduction

In Chapter 1 we discussed the importance of practitioners becoming critical and self aware. A reflective practitioner will be looking closely at their professional practice, asking "what is the best way of doing this?", or "why do we do it this way?". It may be that a practitioner acts on the basis of tradition or an intuitive "knowing in action" which derives from experience (Schon, 1983) but a reflective practitioner will wish to inform their decision.

The shift from an occupation to a profession which has taken place in nursing and health promotion, is characterized by an increased focus on research as the profession attempts to establish its own body of knowledge. There is considerable pressure for all health and welfare practitioners to be research-based and be aware of studies relevant to their practice. Practitioners may be aware that research forms the base of their practice but could not pinpoint any specific findings. Couchman and Dawson (1995) suggest that this may be because practitioners are not aware of the relevant research journals or they may not have the access or the opportunity to keep up to date with research. They may also be sceptical of the value of research because it is difficult to institute any change in their practice.

Example

The following practitioners when asked to identify research that had made an impact on them were all able to cite a particular study:

Jackie, a nurse

"I can remember Doll and Peto's (1981) work on smoking. It didn't have a huge impact at first but all our journals started to be full of the links between smoking and early death."

Judy, a health visitor

"I remember reading about Brown and Harris' (1978) study on depression in women. What struck me really for the first time, was that it wasn't a matter of individual pathology but social isolation. It did change my practice – I looked for ways to provide social support rather than just coping mechanisms."

Jenny, a Health Promotion Specialist

"The works of Tim Lang and Issy Cole-Hamilton in the 1980s on the problems of healthy eating on a low income were really important for us (Cole-Hamilton and Lang, 1986). We were working to government guidelines from the NACNE and COMA reports and it made us re-think how blithely we were putting forward these recommendations."

Jane, a teacher and counsellor

"The Kinsey Report (1948, 1953) has probably had the greatest long-term impact. It has been fundamental in raising our awareness about sexual identity – that not all young people we see are heterosexual and that some might be extremely anxious."

Yet few practitioners see research as an integral component of their practice. It is seen as "out there", separate from the knowledge base that informs practice, which is often received wisdom passed on from practitioner to student.

A practitioner may, however, have a whole host of questions relating to their practice. The Macmillan nurse may want to know why women choose not to come for mammography screening. The Health Promotion Specialist may want to know whether a safety education programme for young children has made any difference to the accident rate. A midwife might want to find out the needs of prospective fathers from the antenatal services. If we see research as providing the information on which to plan and carry out interventions, then research ceases to be seen as a remote activity but becomes an extension of everyday work.

It is likely that your responses to the Reflection point fell into three broad areas:

R What do you think of when you hear the term "research"?

- Methods – the tools used for collecting information, e.g. questionnaires, interviews, experiments, case studies.
- Design – the way in which an enquiry is set up, e.g. the nature and recruitment of the sample.
- Methodology – the principles that underpin the research.

This chapter aims to help you reflect on the methodology of research for health promotion and to consider what distinguishes research in this area. It looks at the social context in which research for health promotion takes place and the kind of information that informs health promotion practice. It is not a tool kit to make you a better researcher. Some excellent texts are recommended at the end of the chapter that can provide guided tours of research methods and the fine tuning in using particular methods. Above all, being a researcher involves doing research and "getting your hands dirty"; it cannot be learnt from a book.

What is research?

Health promotion is based on theories about what influences people's health and what then constitutes an effective intervention or strategy to improve health. Such theories are based on research. The term "research" may be used to describe any systematic information-gathering activity which is used to describe, explain or explore an issue in order to generate new knowledge.

D What do you think distinguishes research from everyday finding out about things that interest you?

Research is:

- the investigation of the real world;
- informed by values about the issue under investigation;
- follows agreed practices and is sensitive to ethical implications;
- asks meaningful questions;
- is systematic and rigorous.

There are several ways in which research informs health promotion and contributes to its development. It may help, for example, to determine priorities for action from a seemingly endless list of possibilities. Epidemiological research or a needs assessment exercise may be the starting point for deciding which issues should be tackled. Evaluative research may determine the effectiveness or acceptability of particular interventions. A research audit may examine which resources and systems are in place for the purpose of improving the performance of an organization or project. Research can also support, challenge or generate new theory. The studies cited by the practitioners on page 26 are all examples of research which contributes to the body of knowledge informing health promotion.

Research has achieved a much higher profile in Health Authorities and health organizations in recent years. Policy and service provision is expected to be based on research and practitioners are being exhorted to base their practice on evidence. The Department of Health has called for reliable research which evaluates practice and procedures as well as the knowledge gained from individual professional experience (DoH, 1993). Evidence-based practice is about effectiveness. A practitioner needs to know for example, whether sex education in schools delays sexual activity (Peersman *et al.*, 1996) or which smoking cessation initiatives are most successful (Reid *et al.*, 1995). The impetus for the development of Research and Development strategies is almost inevitably a budget one – what is a cost-effective intervention? In Chapter 3 we look at the particular problems this poses for health promotion in staking its claim for effectiveness against clinical interventions which may bring more immediate and measurable benefits. It is thus possible to distinguish between research **of** health promotion which looks at whether health promotion has an impact and research **for** health promotion which informs the practice of health promotion.

Research for health promotion derives primarily from public health and epidemiology. Epidemiology has been described as "completing the clinical picture" (Last, 1994:119). It is concerned with the pattern of diseases in a population. By discovering those groups with high rates of disease and those with low rates it is possible to identify the distinctive features of each group in terms of their environment or lifestyle and which might be associated with their likelihood of disease.

The uses of epidemiology (adapted from Ashton, 1994)

- **To observe the effects of social factors on health** – e.g. linking the rise in the number of cars on the road with the incidence of asthma.
- **To provide a "map" of the distribution and size of health problems in the population** – e.g. infant mortality being distributed unequally among social classes.
- **To estimate the risks to an individual of suffering disease** – e.g. the risks of a woman becoming infected with HIV from having unprotected sex with a male partner who is HIV-positive.
- **To assess the operation of services and the extent to which they meet the population's needs** – e.g. the take-up rate for the breast cancer screening programme and the effect on breast cancer incidence and outcomes.

- **Cross-sectional studies to determine prevalence or patterns of conditions or behaviours in populations or groups at one point in time** – e.g. Allied Dunbar Fitness Survey (Sports Council/HEA, 1992)
- **Case–control studies to investigate the causes of a condition by comparing a group with the condition with a control group** – e.g. an investigation into "Gulf War syndrome" will compare a group of soldiers who fought in the Gulf with a matched group who did not, to see if "Gulf War syndrome" symptoms arise disproportionately in the Gulf soldiers. Particular factors affecting the Gulf soldiers, such as exposure to chemicals would then be investigated to determine their possible contribution to symptoms.
- **Cohort or longitudinal studies to observe a group over time to see if there is any association between particular behaviours or characteristics and patterns of disease** – e.g. The Whitehall 2 study of 10,000 civil servants looks at different employment grades and their incidence of ill-health (Brunner, 1996).
- **Randomized control trial which compares a group who experience an intervention with a similar control group who do not** – e.g. Stanford Heart Disease Prevention Programme 1972–80 looked at the risk factors for Coronary Heart Disease among three communities in the USA. One community received intensive health education through the mass media and one-to-one advice; one community received a mass media campaign; the third control group received no intervention (Maccoby et al., 1977).

The examples above have formed the basis of much health promotion work. The Stanford study has been extremely influential in exposing the limitations of mass media campaigns without interpersonal feedback. The Whitehall study has, since its inception in 1978, reminded practitioners of the influence of social factors as risk factors for Coronary Heart Disease. On the basis of the Allied Dunbar survey, which revealed the sedentary habits of the majority of the British public, a major campaign was launched to build exercise into people's lives.

Epidemiology is thus undoubtedly useful. But it should not be thought of as providing the only information health promoters require. Its findings, as with all research, need to be interpreted within the specific theoretical framework in which it is grounded. The particular use of theory will depend on the paradigm or school of thought in which the researcher is working. When we look at the different methodologies used in research we are also looking at different disciplines – either an attempt to explain phenomena following the procedures of natural science or an attempt to understand the world from the point of view of the people in it. Epidemiology reflects the dominance of the medical science paradigm. This approach seeks to identify the risk factors of disease and is informed by a belief that research needs to be objective and scientific.

Positivist and interpretive paradigms

The dominant research tradition in health care derives from a positivist approach which uses the methods and principles of the natural sciences. It claims that there are phenomena or "facts" which are real and can be studied.

In apparent contrast, the interpretive tradition aims to explore and describe the meaning of phenomena as experienced and perceived by the individual. The tradition derives from the social sciences' concern to understand the subjective meaning of human experience.

Positivism is associated with quantitative research methods – the gathering of "hard" data which can be quantified in some way. Quantitative research attempts to measure aspects of a situation and to explain any differences in these variables between groups or over time. Quantitative research tests a hypothesis which is a suggested explanation of why differences occur. The experiment is the main method. In experimental studies one aspect in two matched groups is varied to see if it makes any difference to the result. Any difference can then be attributed to that variable. In research involving people and their lives, it is impossible to control for all the factors which may influence outcomes. People are not isolated from each other and it may also be impossible to avoid the control group being "contaminated" by contact with those who have received an intervention. For example, evaluation of the Heartbeat Wales programme to reduce Coronary Heart Disease became impossible once the control group in England also had access to a CHD prevention programme launched in England.

The interpretive tradition is associated with qualitative research methods which are more about "coming to know" the ways in which an issue is perceived by the people whom it affects. Thoughts, feelings and meanings are real phenomena which can be studied by the researcher. Through methods such as interviews, observation and case studies the researcher can come to understand the perspective of the participants. In contrast to quantitative methods, there is no assumption about what are the important issues which are then confirmed or disproved. Instead qualitative methods are inductive. Plausible explanations for people's views and experiences are induced from the mass of data these methods can generate. This approach has also been called "grounded theory" (Glaser and Strauss, 1986) because the theory is grounded in and emerges from real life experience.

If we use the example of research into sexual health we can see how different paradigms or schools of thought determine what is to be studied. Most research into the spread of HIV/AIDS has been concerned with discovering the incidence, prevalence and distribution of HIV in the population over time. By comparing the proportion of infected people engaging in different risk activities, attempts are made to correlate risk of infection with behaviour. This knowledge can be used in the targeting and design of health education messages. Epidemiologists can also evaluate the effectiveness of health promotion activities by charting rates of HIV infection against interventions.

D What contribution do you think qualitative research could make to HIV prevention?

Gary Dowsett who designed research programmes for the WHO Global Programme on AIDS has commented on the need for more close-focus research which looks at contexts and social situations in which people make sexual decisions:

> "Utilising precious research resources to maximise the measurement of HIV infection and AIDS in any one country will not greatly enhance the prevention and care/support response. A less exact and more general idea of HIV/AIDS prevalence/incidence will, when coupled with well-theorised understanding of sexual and drug use cultures or contexts, offer far more useful starting points for action than all the surveillance data in the world" (Dowsett, 1995).

Quantitative and qualitative research derive from different epistemological perspectives or views about the nature of knowledge and so are often presented as diametrically opposed. The table below summarizes the two philosophically divergent positions.

Table 2.1 *The differences between quantitative and qualitative research*

	Quantitative	Qualitative
Paradigm	Positivism	Interpretive
Epistemological base	Science	Humanities
Researcher's role	Objectivity and detachment	Subjectivity and engagement
Aim	To progress towards the truth	To understand multiple realities
Purpose	To understand causality	To interpret
Method or strategy	To isolate and study discrete variables	To understand the issue in context
Presentation	Quantification	Meanings
Contribution to theory	Falsification (to disprove hypothesis) Generalization	Grounded theory (theory emerges from the data) Understanding complexity

In recent years this apparent divide between these research traditions has been disputed. Bryman (1988) for example, claims such differences are more debated in the heads of philosophers and scientists than found in practice by researchers. Many texts adopt an eclectic approach to research with "horses for courses" being the byword (Robson, 1993). Most health issues are so complex that different methods are suitable for different tasks and one method may illuminate or inform another.

Those using quantitative methods are often advised that good practice is to inform their study with exploratory qualitative research. Different methods can, in addition, tap multiple realities and thus arrive at more valid findings. Triangulation refers to the use of multiple methods as a means of increasing validity. "Triangulation in surveying is a method of finding out where something is by getting a fix from two or more places. Analogously, Denzin (1988) suggested that this might be done in social research by using multiple methods, investigators or theories" (Robson, 1993:290).

Despite such arguments about interdependence, we claim that there remains an epistemological divide. Qualitative research is seen as subjective and lacking rigour because the researcher doesn't just observe but is directly involved with the subjects of the study. Findings are not seen to be generalizable as samples are usually too small and unrepresentative to be statistically valid. Because qualitative research doesn't require any particular statistical expertise, it is often assumed that anyone with a modicum of interpersonal skills can do it (Boulton and Fitzpatrick, 1994). Quantitative research, on the other hand is seen as abstract, requiring special expertise and unrelated to the social world of the individuals which it studies.

What counts as research?

A ctivity

Why do a high proportion of women stop breast feeding within two weeks of their return home after delivery?

Consider the following two research studies and decide which of the two studies is more likely to get research funding and why.

Which of the two studies is more likely to get published in a nursing, midwifery or medical journal?

Study 1

Two groups of new mothers from Newtown Hospital are compared. In one group are women who are breast feeding at 8 weeks and in the other group are mothers who stopped breast feeding within 2 weeks. The two groups are compared using tests for statistical significance to see if there are any specific variables that discriminate between the two groups and which might explain the difference.

Study 2
A series of in-depth interviews with a small sample of new mothers at Newtown hospital about their perceptions and feelings about breast feeding.

Although this is a very simple example, you probably concluded immediately that the first study would be more likely to get funding and to be published. Researchers seeking funding often find that there is a methodological status hierarchy whereby qualitative research is deemed less legitimate than quantitative biomedical or epidemiological research (Pope and Mays, 1993). When seeking to get work published, the format many journals require – of hypothesis or question, method, results and discussion – reflects the type of research which will be deemed acceptable.

Funding for health promotion research may come from health authorities or the Health Education Authority or research bodies such as the Economic and Social Science Research Council or occasionally commercial organizations with a research arm such as the Wellcome Trust. The shift towards consumerism and accountability in the NHS has served to increase interest in qualitative research which gives people a voice. Nevertheless it is still difficult to get recognition for the qualitative work which informs health promotion. Most Research and Development strategies do not explicitly include health promotion as a category and health promotion is interpreted within the dominant preventive medical framework; in other words, epidemiological studies of particular diseases, studies on individual lifestyle determinants or the prevention of specific conditions through screening, surveillance or immunization. Until now, the areas which have been designated as having utility and relevance are those relating to "Health of the Nation" or health gain. In line with the theme of evidence-based practice, the criteria for research projects in the NHS do not cater for exploratory projects but focus on reviewing effectiveness. The tradition of high status quantitative research presents a dilemma for health promoters who are caught between emulating quantitative research or promoting qualitative research with all the problems of credibility and authority this entails.

Feminists have drawn attention to the need to identify the values of the institutions in which research takes place. Doyal (1995) argues that the priorities and techniques, particularly of biomedical research, reflects the male domination of the profession. She suggests that non-reproductive conditions affecting women such as osteoporosis or incontinence get ignored and other health issues are seen as a "male" problem. For example, an important study which demonstrated the effectiveness of daily aspirin consumption in preventing cardiovascular disease did not include any women in its sample (Freedman and Maine, 1993).

R Can you think of an example of research relating to issues of interest or significance to a particular group which has not been taken up or funded?

The definition of the issue to be studied, the methods used to carry out the research, the interpretation of the results and the dissemination of findings all reflect the way in which health promotion is perceived. So when we think about research for health promotion we need to think about what sort of information we need and what paradigm we are working in.

Research for health promotion

Scott-Samuel (1989) has argued that what health promotion requires is a social epidemiology which is:

- subjective;
- collective;
- participative and non-expertist.

The principles of the World Health Organization Health For All strategy (WHO, 1985) acknowledge that health is a relative concept to which people attach different meanings. Lay views of health and illness must be taken into account when trying to promote health. The WHO defines health promotion as enabling people to increase control over their health and the factors influencing their health. This demands research which enables the subjects of any study to be active participants in it and for the research to achieve change for that community.

Lay knowledge

Epidemiology, upon which public health knowledge has depended, rests upon the concept of disease. It tends to focus on the causes and risks of dying or becoming ill. What is lacking is an understanding of the subjective experience of health and illness. Medicine depends on the ability to diagnose – that there is some sign and indication of pathology which takes precedence over the individual experience of ill-health or disease. Yet the current commitment of the NHS to identifying population and community needs demands a form of inquiry which describes health as ordinary people perceive it. The WHO recognized this a decade ago when they stated that "more emphasis should be laid on qualitative methods of observation, namely, those that allow lay people to define a problem and its solution from their own viewpoint" (WHO, 1986:121). Milburn (1996) observes how the conundrum for health promotion of the lack of relationship between people's knowledge, attitudes and behaviour would be illuminated by knowing more about the meanings and socio-cultural contexts which influence behaviour.

D Take a health issue with which you are familiar. How might lay concepts of health and illness help to develop culturally appropriate health promotion practice around this issue?

Research has shown that people have their own lay epidemiology and understanding of the causes of ill-health which is influenced by:

- beliefs about "candidacy" (the image of the kind of person that suffers from, for example, heart disease);
- beliefs about luck and fate in relation to illness;
- how social networks develop and affirm ideas about "candidacy";
- beliefs about the life cycle and personal assessments of what it means to be healthy at different ages (Davison *et al.*, 1991, 1992).

The ways in which researchers find out about people's ways of seeing and talking about illness vary from the large-scale survey (Blaxter, 1990) to studies from an ethnographic or biographical perspective. Cornwell's (1984) case study of a group of families in the East End of London gives not only a fascinating insight into the ideas and concepts about health, illness and health services but also shows how health is integral to people's lives. Cornwell states that her study "has more in common with social anthropology than with other disciplines in the social sciences, in so far as the emphasis in social anthropology is all the time on the whole and on the links between apparently discrete areas of social life" (Cornwell, 1984:1).

Hilary Graham's studies of the lives of working class women uses data from open-ended accounts recorded by researchers and the personal views of women recorded in letters, diaries, and pictures. This commentary on how women represent themselves and make sense of their lives is presented in contrast to official and survey data which tends to "exclude and misrepresent those most affected by disadvantage and discrimination" (Graham, 1993:34). Williams and Popay (1994:122) suggest that lay knowledge represents a challenge to medicine "because it means taking subjectivity seriously rather than seeing it as an impediment to understanding". One of the claims of scientific knowledge is that it is objective and impartial. Lay knowledge represents another way of knowing. Although unrepresentative in a statistical sense, studies of lay beliefs do draw upon ideas that are general and shared. They thus present other discourses which need to be acknowledged and which compete with and contest the truth-claims of scientific knowledge.

D

Consider the following examples where lay knowledge has suggested new avenues for research, which had hitherto been ignored by scientific research:

- Links between child hyperactivity and food additives.
- Links between the seasons and sense of well-being.
- The efficacy of complementary therapies.

Can you think of any more examples?

Williams and Popay also see lay knowledge as representing a political challenge to the power of experts to determine the way in which issues for policy are defined. The following piece of research came about through intense media pressure which in turn came about because of pressure from ordinary people who thought there was some connection between their ill-health and an external factor and that research would substantiate something they felt they already knew. Yet the research study used large-scale experimental designs with matched control groups. Why? Because such research is deemed to be scientific, objective and explanatory.

Example

Radiation and leukaemia

In one study 97 cases of childhood and adolescent leukaemia and lymphoma diagnosed in West Cumbria between 1950 and 1985 were matched with 1001 controls. The study showed an association between the father's radiation dose prior to conception of the child and the child's risk of leukaemia. The study has been subject to enormous scrutiny both in its data collection process and the analysis of the data. It has been cited in a long court case brought against British Nuclear Fuels, the owners of Sellafield (previously called Windscale) nuclear processing plant in Cumbria. (Source: Gardner *et al.*, 1990).

One of the challenges facing health promotion research is to discover what people mean by health or well-being. A central plank of health promotion is that it is based on a concept of positive health, rather than merely the absence of disease or infirmity. Researching positive health is still in its infancy. Most attempts to tap into this area have focused on defining indicators of well-being, the best known being the Nottingham Health Profile. The questions used to form the basis of this assessment are, however, generally couched in negative terms focusing on the absence of symptoms, e.g. "Have you felt tired this week?" Antonovsky (1984) has highlighted some of the limitations of the "pathogenic" paradigm which looks for the causes of disease. He argues that the focus on eliminating disease has led to the identification of risk groups and ignored those aspects which enable some people to cope with disease. Antonovsky calls instead for a "salutogenic" model of health which would seek to identify "symptoms of wellness".

D How would using a "salutogenic" model of health affect the kind of research carried out around specific issues, e.g. smoking?

Research using a salutogenic model of health might for example, identify low income groups with very low rates of smoking, e.g. Asian women, and seek to understand how such groups resist the adoption of smoking as a coping mechanism.

Participative research

Research from whatever paradigm is often seen as "expert" knowledge. It is produced by and for other experts and can be intimidating and inaccessible to the lay person. There are numerous studies which would be of immediate interest to the public but their findings are not made available.

In many cases research does not enter the public domain unless it is picked up by the media. Anne Diamond, a television presenter who lost a baby from Sudden Infant Death Syndrome (SIDS) in 1991, successfully highlighted research which showed that the number of deaths from SIDS were halved in New Zealand through a national campaign to lay babies to sleep on their backs.

Yet one of the core principles of health promotion, according to the World Health Organization (1986) is that people have a right and duty to participate in the planning of their health care. If research forms the basis for this, then people also have a right to be active and equal participants in that research process and its dissemination.

Research typically involves an expert researcher and passive subjects. Empowering research attempts to shift the balance of power by acknowledging and valuing the participants. This can easily become a principle to be espoused through the use of ethical principles of procedure or non-directive, qualitative methods. However, the best intentions to avoid hierarchical relations of power can be subverted by the practice of research itself which is automatically "other" to the participants and which mediates the voice and experiences of participants whilst presenting their data as authentic and true. Feminist research sees the extent to which participants determine the direction of the study and are involved in the analysis and dissemination of the findings as key issues to be addressed (Bowles and Duelli Klein, 1983).

The research relationship is a power relationship and it is relatively easy for researchers to assume control over the research participants who may have very different expectations and construe the research setting in a different way.

D Why do you think the findings of studies on the following issues are not generally known?

- Can eating beef lead to Creutzfeldt Jakob disease?
- Does the Hib vaccine protect against meningitis?
- Is a glass or two of red wine a day a protection against coronary heart disease?

E xample

Bristol Cancer Help Centre

In the late 1980s 334 women attending the Bristol Cancer Help Centre took part in a clinical trial comparing their treatment which combined complementary therapies and traditional chemotherapy and radiography with the conventional treatment of women at the Royal Marsden Hospital and two district general hospitals. All the women were aged less than 70 and had a single invasive primary cancer of the breast. The study appeared to show that women with breast cancer in the control group who were free of metastases at the time of the study were nearly three times as likely to survive as women in the Bristol group; in other words women would be better off receiving conventional treatment. Almost inevitably a study which produced such clear findings on an issue of great concern meant that the research design was heavily scrutinized and called into question (Bagenal *et al.*, 1990).

The example is cited as an example of research in which the participants had no control and the women ended up publically objecting to its design and findings. They felt that it supported a dominant medical agenda and reflected the scepticism with which complementary therapies are viewed. The women at Bristol Cancer Help Centre felt strongly that a clinical trial was inappropriate to evaluate its work and that their health experience was not taken into account.

Williams and Popay (1994) have shown how research can be used by communities themselves to attract attention to a health issue of concern. They describe the way in which the people of Camelford in Cornwall systematically gathered evidence of the effects on health from their contaminated water supply. Their experience is an illustration of the way in which vested interests can control research findings and how this can be challenged by people becoming active researchers themselves.

E xample	In 1988 a lorry accidentally tipped 20 tonnes of aluminium sulfate into the treated water supply of the people of Camelford in North Cornwall. Local people organized themselves and carefully monitored the health effects of the incident. Their evidence was presented to an independent expert group set up by the Department of Health. The Clayton Committee refuted the local evidence claiming that it had not been collected in a systematic manner and was not representative of the whole population. The report concluded that "in our view it is not possible to attribute the very real current health complaints to the toxic effects of the incident inasmuch as they are the consequence of the sustained anxiety naturally felt by many people".
Camelford and "lay epidemiology"	

Although the people of Camelford knew they were experiencing ill-health, their evidence was put down to hysteria fanned by the media. It was not given credence when compared to the technical, toxicological and clinical measurements of a panel of scientific experts (Williams and Popay, 1994).

Participative research involves working in partnership with the subjects of the research. Research should be seen as an exchange – those who take part should get something from the exchange. Involving participants in the research design and planning can involve complex negotiations and slow down the progress of a project. Giving control over the findings can be similarly time-consuming and dispiriting if it is perceived that the research is not of direct benefit. But as McKie and Gregory assert the beneficiaries of research should always be its participants:

> "directly the results may feed back to them in the form of information and advice offered by the practitioner within the consultation or care process, or in the form of health education and promotion. Indirectly, benefit may be obtained through the improved and extended knowledge gained by the practitioners and policy makers responsible for the design, construction and process of a specific service" (McKie and Gregory, 1996:260).

Social research

Social research is the term used here to describe research which seeks to explore the context in which health decisions are made. In the medical/psychological paradigm, health needs become related to known biomedical risk factors, and collective problems become individualized and related to health behaviours such as smoking, drinking or diet. Gantley (1994) describes research into the causes of Sudden Infant Death Syndrome (SIDS) which suggested that epidemiological analysis should identify risk factors deemed modifiable so that a health education programme could be directed towards individual parents. She goes on to say that socio-economic factors such as social class and educational level were not considered, although there have been suggestions that in countries with specific policies to reduce poverty and inequalities in health there has been a reduction in the incidence of SIDS.

Although there is now a mass of evidence documenting the social and economic dimension of health and illness (e.g. Blackburn, 1991; Benzeval et al., 1995) such research has been disputed during the 18 years of Conservative administration. The Department of Health acknowledged that there are significant social variations in health but refused to acknowledge the relationship between income and health. The focus of research was into socio-behavioural factors and studies of the factors influencing access to and uptake of health and social care (DoH, 1995). A review of the evidence linking inequalities with health was one of the first tasks of the Labour government in 1997.

As the official neglect of health inequalities research under the Conservative government shows, research is a powerful tool which takes place in a political context. The political acceptability of research findings is often more important than its quality in determining the profile and level of publicity of research.

Example

Housing and health

The health impact of housing, and in particular the link between damp housing and respiratory disease, had been largely ignored until a study by Hunt and others in 1986. Hunt suggests that there were two reasons for this:

- The unfashionable nature of the topic and its potentially political implications.
- The way in which the topic was fragmented among different professional groups (allergies from mould being the province of doctors, Environmental Health being concerned with dampness, the identification of mould being done by building surveyors and microbiologists and the structural problems which give rise to damp being the responsibility of architects).

The ill-health of people living in damp housing was thus seen as the consequence of poverty and individual behaviour such as smoking and boiling nappies and potatoes rather than as a consequence of mould in the air and on the walls which her study confirmed as a major cause of ill-health (Hunt, 1993).

An international workshop of physicians, researchers and health practitioners who met to debate the future of public health research called for a multidisciplinary research framework to overcome the limitations of studies in which issues are framed solely within a biomedical model. The Leeds Declaration called for health promotion research to be methodologically eclectic and recognize the contribution of different disciplines. In the call for a re-focus upstream away from individual risks, the document acknowledges the ways in which the social sciences in particular can help to illuminate the contexts and structures in which ill-health originates (Nuffield Institute, 1993).

ctivity

The Leeds Declaration (extracts)
- Research is needed to explore the factors which keep some people healthy despite their living in the most adverse circumstances.
- Lay people are experts and experts are lay people – lay knowledge about health needs, health service priorities and health outcomes should be central to public health research.
- The experimental model is an inadequate gold standard for guiding research into public health problems.
- A plurality of methods is required to address the multiple dimensions of public health problems.
- Not all health data can be represented in numbers – qualitative data has an important role to play in public health research.
- There is nothing inherently "soft" about qualitative methods or "hard" about quantitative methods – both require rigorous application in appropriate contexts and hard thinking about difficult problems.

How would you assess the:

■   usefulness;
■   practicality;
■   ethical and political acceptability of these principles for action?

Are there any additional principles you would add?

The practitioner-researcher

So far in this chapter we have looked at the nature of the research which informs health promotion and how this illustrates a bio-medical framework. In the previous section we called for research which echoes the principles of the Health For All movement. Research for health promotion would focus on:

■   health not illness;
■   its social determinants;

and would be carried out in ways which were empowering for participants.

Alongside this, practitioners need to become critical consumers of research, knowing the research in their area and being able to evaluate it with confidence. Research may challenge current practice – at what point should research be used to justify a change in practice?

R   What examples can you think of in your area of work where a long-held practice has been changed. Can you attribute the change to research findings?

Examples from midwifery and health visiting might include the change in advice to parents about the sleeping position of babies who should not be laid down on their fronts; or the abandonment of enemas and pubic shaving during delivery; or the introduction of postnatal support.

Research can challenge taken for granted assumptions and therefore being research-minded is a crucial part of reflective practice. But it is also important to be critical: how does one decide which evidence is sufficiently convincing to influence practice? Because this is difficult, and because knowledge is never a given but is always changing, practitioners often resort to their "knowing-in action" and ignore new findings. There may also be a delay in the diffusion and adoption of interventions because they are not widely known. The publication of effectiveness reviews and meta-analyses (see Chapter 3) may help to diffuse knowledge but they need to be more user-friendly and adopt wider criteria than the randomized controlled trial as the "gold standard" if they are to help practitioners directly.

D

What is health promotion advice about saturated fat in the diet?

- Substitute with low fat products.
- Eat more fibre to reduce cholesterol.
- Diet is not the main risk factor for coronary heart disease.
- Try to reduce stress instead.

On what evidence would you base your advice?
The evidence for each of these pieces of advice is far from clear. Low fat products involve a chemical processing, the effects of which are not fully known. Fibre does reduce cholesterol but it is not known how this occurs or how much fibre intake is necessary. The relative contribution of dietary fats, stress or genetic history as risk factors for CHD is not known. (See Chapter 10 for discussion on approaches to CHD prevention.)

Most training courses for health and welfare practitioners now include research awareness and skills and alert students to ways in which research studies can lack rigour. Common problems include making claims that are not substantiated by the data, or claiming findings from exploratory studies can be generalized, or providing selective data to support a particular point of view. It is also important to be able to identify when research has been conducted rigorously. For quantitative research, rigour is achieved through representative samples which ensures that findings can be generalized. Statistical manipulation of the data must be appropriate for the kind and quality of data obtained. For qualitative research, rigour is achieved through being systematic and open in the methods used and applying critical reflection to the research process. Rigorous qualitative research achieves relatability; or the discovery of insights which can be used in similar situations.

In the following chapter we look at the very strict criteria which are used to classify studies of effective health promotion interventions. For practitioners, reading about research is a key component of developing research expertise both substantively and practically. Making a reasoned judgement about the value of a research study takes skill and practice but analysing strengths and weaknesses in the work of others helps practitioners in the design of their own studies. The questions to ask when evaluating published research can be put into a checklist (Figure 2.1).

Published papers are usually refereed by external reviewers in the field but this does not guarantee that the research is trustworthy. There is also a mass of needs assessment and evaluation studies which practitioners carry out routinely but which are not published and so remain invisible. It is important that practitioners do share their findings and experiences by bringing them into the public domain through reports, articles, and conference papers. In this way

Research problem
■ How relevant is the issue to the "real world"?
■ Does it challenge or amplify existing ideas on the issue?
■ Does it have a clear theoretical framework?
■ What particular questions does the study try to answer?
■ Are the objectives clearly stated?

Influences on the research
■ How does the background or experience of the researchers, and the source of funding influence the nature of the research?

Method
■ Is the choice of method suitable to the issue?
■ Has the study been conducted with control and rigour?
■ Are the size, composition, selection and representativeness of the sample clearly stated?
■ How valid are the instruments (do they measure what they are intended to measure)?
■ How reliable are the instruments (would similar results be obtained if the study was repeated)?
■ How were the instruments developed? Was there a pilot study?

Results
■ Are the results clear and understandable?
■ Are the data presented relevant to the aims?
■ How were the data analysed and presented?
■ Are any statistical tests appropriate to the kind of data gathered? (e.g. to show confidence levels and whether the results could have arisen by chance).

Conclusions
■ Do the conclusions follow from the data?
■ Is the study critical of the methodology employed?
■ What light do the findings shed on the background theory? Are alternative explanations possible?
■ Does the study make recommendations for practice and are these justified by the research as presented?

Ethical issues
■ Has the study paid attention to issues of confidentiality and consent?
■ Are the values of the researcher stated and discussed?
■ In whose interests is the research conducted?

Figure 2.1 *Checklist for evaluating published research (adapted from Couchman and Dawson, 1995 and Rawson, unpublished).*

the body of knowledge and theory about the relatively new field of health promotion can be developed.

A practitioner-researcher is someone who, in addition to their work, carries out systematic enquiry relevant to their work. Apart from the few posts which are designated as having these joint roles, for the majority doing research is an additional responsibility. Practitioners are in a valuable position to carry out research with their knowledge, contacts and position within an organization, but carrying out research as a practitioner does have particular difficulties:

- lack of time;
- lack of funding;
- lack of expertise in research design and methods;
- lack of confidence;
- lack of credibility within the organization that small-scale research could offer anything more than existing knowledge;
- research not being perceived as relevant or a priority for the setting in which it would take place;
- the need to negotiate with other staff or clients;
- ethical considerations about the ways in which research can impact on those involved.

As well as being a critical consumer of research, there is an increasing emphasis on practitioners being accountable for their practice and therefore engaging in reviews of its effectiveness. They are called upon to demonstrate the health gain from any intervention and to base decision making on research. This brings practitioners back full circle to the medical paradigm and the assumption that research is non-problematic, objective and can provide an answer. In this and the following chapter we have argued that research for health promotion needs to go beyond this paradigm and take a broader view developing and using research in accordance with its aims and values.

Conclusion

Health promotion has inherited a positivist tradition which has tended to mystify research and made it seem remote and difficult. Practitioners view research as a separate activity which they tend not to get involved with or use as a tool to improve practice. Yet the principles of research are ones that all practitioners can use – being aware of the way in which an issue is being defined and the philosophical principles which underpin the approach to its study, the need to reflect on theory and the ability to scrutinize and analyse available information. This practice of enquiry is an addition to the kind of knowing that an experienced practitioner already has and it is a "means of organising common sense and intuitive problem-solving so as to guard against some of their short-comings" (Robson, 1993:461).

In addition to the argument that research is a tool for practice there is also the view that health promotion is dependent on research. As a newly emerging profession, research provides the epistemological base for health promotion. It is crucial that the nature of this research is sympathetic to the aims and values of health promotion. Hence the calls for participative research directed towards the social determinants of health and for qualitative research which seeks to understand people's health experience.

Further discussion

■ To what extent can health promotion research be translated into action and policy?

■ What importance do you give to research in your work? Should your practice be more research linked? If so, how could you do this?

Recommended reading

■ Couchman W and Dawson J (1995) *Nursing and health care research: a practical guide*, London, Scutari.
A basic introduction to research methods which includes activities and exercises to develop skills.

■ McConway, K (ed.) (1994) *Studying Health and Disease*, Buckingham, Open University Press.

■ Unwin N, Carr S, Leeson J with Pless-Mulloli T (1996) *Public Health and Epidemiology*, Buckingham, Open University Press.
Two textbooks which provide an introduction to the kinds of health data that are collected and how they might be analysed.

■ Popay J and Williams G (eds) (1994) *Researching the People's Health*, London, Routledge.
An interesting collection of contributions from social researchers which looks at the relationship between lay knowledge and expert knowledge.

■ Abramson J (1997) "Epidemiology to be taken with care", Sidell M, Jones L, Katz J and Peberdy A (eds) *Debates and Dilemmas in Promoting Health: A Reader*, pp. 143–156, Basingstoke, MacMillan/Open University.

■ Tannahill A (1992) in Bunton R and Macdonald G (eds) *Health Promotion: Disciplines and Diversity*, pp. 86–107, London, Routledge.
These chapters both argue that health promoters should have a grasp of epidemiology but also suggest that it should not be the only information required.

■ Robson C (1993) *Real World Research*, Oxford, Blackwell.
One of the most recent and comprehensive guides to research methods. It is an excellent guide for both new and more experienced researchers.

■ Wilson Barnett J and Macleod Clark J (eds) (1993) *Research in health promotion and nursing*, Basingstoke, Macmillan.
A collection of empirical research on health promotion within nursing practice. The studies vary in size and methodologies and illustrate some of the areas deemed important for nursing research.

References

Antonovsky A (1993) "The sense of coherence as a determinant of health", in Beattie A *et al.* (eds) *Health and Wellbeing: A Reader*, Basingstoke, MacMillan/Open University.

Ashton J (ed.) (1994) *The epidemiological imagination*, Buckingham, Open University Press.

Bagenal FS, Easton DF, Harris E, Chilvers CED and McElwain TJ (1990) "Survival of patients with breast cancer attending Bristol Cancer Help Centre", *Lancet*, **336**, 606–10.

Benzeval M, Judge K and Whitehead M (1995) *Tackling inequalities in health*, London, Kings Fund.

Blackburn C (1991) *Poverty and Health: working with families*, Buckingham, Open University Press.

Blaxter M (1990) *Health and lifestyles*, London, Tavistock.

Boulton M and Fitzpatrick R (1994) " 'Quality' in qualitative research", *Critical Public Health*, **5**(3), 19–26.

Bowles G and Duelli Klein L (1983) *Theories of Womens Studies*, London, Routledge Kegan Paul.

Brown GW and Harris T (1978) *Social Origins of Depression*, London, Tavistock.

Brunner E (1996) "The social and biological basis of cardiovascular disease in office workers", in Blane D, Brunner E and Wilkinson R (eds), *Health and Social Organisation: Towards a health policy for the 21st century*, London, Routledge.

Bryman A (1988) *Quality and Quantity in Social Research*, London, Unwin Hyman.

Cole-Hamilton I and Lang T (1986) *Tightening belts – a report on the impact of poverty on food*, London, London Food Commission.

Cornwell J (1984) *Hard Earned Lives: accounts of health and illness from East London*, London, Tavistock.

Couchman W and Dawson J (1995) *Nursing and health care research*, 2nd edn, London, Scutari.

Davison C, Davey Smith G and Frankel S (1991) "Lay epidemiology and the Prevention Paradox: the implications of coronary candidacy for health education", *Sociology of Health and Illness*, **13**(1), 1–19.

Davison C, Frankel S and Davey Smith G (1992) "The limits of lifestyle: reassessing 'fatalism' in the popular culture of illness prevention", *Social Science and Medicine*, **34**(6), 675–85.

Denzin N (1988) *The research act: a theoretical introduction to sociological methods*, 3rd edn, New Jersey, Prentice Hall.

Department of Health (1993) *Report of the taskforce on the strategy for research in nursing, midwifery and health visiting*, London, HMSO.

Department of Health (1995) *Variations in health: what can the Department of Health and the NHS do?* London, HMSO.

Doll R and Peto R (1981) *The causes of cancer*, Oxford, Oxford University Press.

Dowsett G (1995) "Focus on HIV/AIDS research", *Healthlines*, **28**, December.

Doyal L (1995) *What makes women sick?* Basingstoke, Macmillan.

Freedman L and Maine D (1993) "Women's mortality: a legacy of neglect", in Koblinsky M, Timyan J and Gay J (eds), *The health of women: a global perspective*, Boulder, Colorado, Westview Press.

Gantley M (1994) "The qualitative and the quantitative: an anthropological perspective on research methods", *Critical Public Health*, **5**(3), 27–32.

Gardner MJ, Snee MP, Hall AJ, Powell CA, Davies S and Terrell JD (1990) "Results of a case control study of leukaemia and lymphoma among young people near Sellafield nuclear plant in West Cumbria", *British Medical Journal*, **300**, 423–29.

Glaser B and Strauss A (1986) *The discovery of grounded theory: strategies for qualitative research*, Chicago, Aldine.

Graham H (1993) *Hardship and Health in Women's Lives*, Hemel Hempstead, Harvester Wheatsheaf.

Hunt SM (1993) "The relationship between research and policy: translating knowledge into action", in Davies JK and Kelly M (eds) *Healthy Cities: research and practice*, London, Routledge.

Kinsey AC, Pomeroy WB and Martin CE (1948) *Sexual behaviour in the human male*, Philadelphia, WB Saunders.

Kinsey AC, Pomeroy WB, Martin CE and Gebhard PH (1953) *Sexual behaviour in the human female*, Philadelphia, WB Saunders.

Last J (1994) "The uses of epidemiology", in Ashton J (ed.) *The epidemiological imagination*, Buckingham, Open University Press.

Maccoby N *et al.* (1977) "Reducing the risk of cardiovascular disease: effects of a community based campaign on knowledge and behaviour", *Journal of Community Health*, **3**, 100–114.

McKie L and Gregory S (1996) "Reflecting on the process and methods of researching women's health", in McKie L (ed.) *Researching Women's Health*, Wiltshire, Quay.

Milburn K (1996) "The importance of lay theorising for health promotion research and practice", *Health promotion International*, **11**(1), 41–47.

Nuffield Institute for Health (1993) *Directions for health: new approaches to population health research and practice. The Leeds Declaration*, cited in Lancet editorial "Population health looking upstream", *Lancet*, **343**, 1994, 429–30.

Peersman G, Oakley A, Oliver S and Thomas J (1996) *Review of effectiveness of sexual health promotion interventions for young people*, Social Science Research Unit, London University Institute of Education.

Pope C and Mays N (1993) Opening the black box: an encounter in the corridors of health services research, *British Medical Journal*, **306**, 315–18.

Reid D, McNeill A and Glynn T (1995) "Reducing the prevalence of smoking in youth: an international review", *Tobacco Control*, **4**, 266–77.

Robson C (1993) *Real World Research: a resource for social scientists and practitioner-researchers*, Oxford, Blackwell.

Schon D (1983) *The reflective practitioner*, London, Temple Smith.

Scott Samuel A (1989) "Building the new public health: a Public Health Alliance and a new social epidemiology", in Martin CJ and McQueen DV (eds) *Readings for a new public health*, Edinburgh, Edinburgh University Press.

Sports Council/HEA (1992) *Allied Dunbar National Fitness Survey*, London, Health Education Authority.

WHO (1985) *Health for All in Europe by the Year 2000*, Copenhagen, WHO.

WHO (1986) "Lifestyles and Health" cited in *Social Science*, **22**, 117–24.

Williams G and Popay J (1994) "Lay knowledge and the privilege of experience", in Gabe J, Kelleher D and Williams G (eds) *Challenging Medicine*, London, Routledge.

3 *Effectiveness and evidence-based practice in health promotion*

Key points

- Effectiveness.
- Evidence-based practice.
- Meta-analysis.
- Deciding *what* to measure:
  - □ medical model;
  - □ educational model;
  - □ behavioural or lifestyles model;
  - □ social model;
  - □ empowerment model.
- Cost-effectiveness.
- *Who* is the audience?

Overview

Recent proposals to make healthcare services more responsive to research evidence rely on agreement as to what determines effectiveness. The previous chapter considered what research for and of health promotion means in practice. This chapter examines the concepts of effectiveness and evidence-based practice in relation to health promotion. Different criteria used to evaluate research evidence are examined and the case is made that health promotion, because of its core principles, should be evaluated in different and complementary ways. Whilst scientific criteria may be appropriate for medical interventions, the more process-oriented objectives of much health promotion work require a range of evaluative criteria, including those drawn from the social sciences as well as medical science.

Introduction

Whether health promotion is effective has always been a key concern for practitioners. For specialist health promotion departments, proving their work is both necessary and effective is vital, as they are competing with other provider trusts for resources. As we saw in Chapter 1, an increasing range of practitioners have a remit for health promotion, but retaining its profile in the context of increased workloads and drives for efficiency savings will be difficult unless there is convincing evidence that health promotion *does* work.

Several organizations, governmental and academic, are engaged in researching the effectiveness of health promotion: NHS Centre for Reviews and Dissemination; Health Education Authority for England; Health Promotion Wales; Health Education Board for Scotland; NHS Regional Research and Development Departments; Social Science

Research Unit based at the Institute of Education, London University; Health Care Evaluation Unit based at the University of Bristol; Health and Behaviour Research Unit based at the University of Edinburgh. Increasingly, evaluation strategies seek to include practitioners and academics in collaborative research.

The worth of health promotion can be assessed according to:

■   effectiveness (the extent to which objectives are met);
■   efficiency (the relative balance of costs to benefits);
■   appropriateness (relevance to need);
■   acceptability (sensitivity and flexibility);
■   equity (equal provision for equal need).

This chapter aims to help health promoters take an active part in the current debate around effectiveness by clarifying the key issues involved. We look first at how to define effectiveness, and note that competing definitions give rise to different ways of assessing effectiveness. We then investigate who constitutes the potential audience for research on effectiveness. Together with the previous chapter, this chapter discusses how health promotion, which lacks the disciplinary status of other areas, can build and improve its practice through research.

Defining effectiveness

| R   What do you understand by "effective health promotion"? |

There is a range of interpretations as to what effectiveness means when applied to health promotion. For some, effectiveness refers to achieving long-term outcomes such as changes in mortality. More commonly, intermediate indicators such as changes in risk factors (e.g. obesity or high blood pressure) are used. Behavioural change is often measured through observation or self reports to determine the effectiveness of health promotion activities. Other definitions of effectiveness include changes in attitudes or knowledge, organizational policy development or legislative and regulatory changes.

As can be seen, deciding what criteria to use to determine effectiveness depends on what are seen as the objectives of health promotion. Chapter 1 highlighted the importance of practitioners being clear about the purpose of health promotion interventions and basing their work on a theoretical understanding.

Practitioners are often required to evaluate the effect of their activities and organizations may evaluate projects with which they are involved. However, many of these evaluations are not carried out with sufficient rigour and remain unpublished. These studies cannot be used with confidence as a base for future practice. This has led to attempts to draw together available evidence in reviews of the effectiveness of health education and health promotion, examples of which are given in Table 3.1.

Table 3.1 *Reviews of the effectiveness of health promotion*

Research Organization	Topic of research	References
The Health Care Evaluation Unit, University of Bristol	Screening for diabetic retinopathy	Bachmann and Nelson, 1996
	Fragile X syndrome	Bredow and Harvey, 1995
	Ovarian cancer	Pearson, 1993
	Antenatal genetic and ultrasound screening	Pearson, 1995, 1994a
	Prostate cancer	HCEU, 1996
	Suicide prevention	Gunnell, 1994
	Skin cancer prevention	Harvey, 1995
	Preconception care	Pearson, 1994b
	Antenatal care	Pearson, 1994c
	Prenatal diagnosis	Richards, 1995
The Health Education Authority, London	Smoking cessation	HEA, 1993a; Buck and Godfrey, 1994
	Prevention of unintentional injuries in childhood and young adolescence	HEA, 1996a
	Coronary heart disease and stroke prevention in older people	HEA, 1996b
	HIV and AIDS prevention	Moody *et al.*, 1991
	Nutrition interventions in primary health care	HEA, 1993b
	The effectiveness of video in health education	Eiser and Eiser, 1996
	The effectiveness of health promotion with young people	HEA, 1996c
	In particular, strategies to reduce alcohol and substance misuse among young people	HEA, 1997a, 1997b
The NHS Centre for Reviews and Dissemination, the University of York	Health service interventions to reduce variations in health	NHS CRD, 1995
	Ethnicity and the health areas of cardiovascular disease, mental health and haemoglobinopathies	NHS CRD, 1996a
The Social Science Research Unit, the Institute of Education, University of London	Sex education	Oakley *et al.*, 1995
Health Promotion Wales	Oral health promotion	Sprod *et al.*, 1996

These studies use meta-analysis to provide a summary of the best research evidence available. Meta-analysis is used to "pool the results of individual studies to produce a weighted average which gives more weight to the more informative studies . . . and less weight to the least informative studies" (NHS CRD, 1996b:48). Meta-analysis sets out methodological criteria which are used to include or exclude research studies. Guidelines are available for the conduct of systematic reviews or meta-analyses of research on effectiveness (NHS CRD, 1996b). Table 3.2 below gives a hierarchy of evidence.

Studies are deemed to have desirable methodological characteristics if:

1. the intervention is described in sufficient detail so that it could be replicated by others;
2. the target audience is fully described;
3. the size and effect of non-respondents is included;
4. there are clear outcomes or health status measurements;
5. these outcomes are compared to baseline measurements undertaken before the intervention.

Meta-analysis typically takes the experimental study as the "gold standard", and large numbers of studies are often excluded because their methodology is deemed to be insufficiently rigorous. This poses a problem for practitioners and researchers alike. If time, effort and resources are being expended on research into effectiveness which is dismissed as unsound, practitioners are losing the opportunity of influencing practice and policy. Whilst it may be argued that meta-analysis is over-committed to a particular model of research (the

D What criteria of methodological validity (aspects of research design which would lead you to be confident that the results are meaningful and generalizable to other populations) would you stipulate if you were conducting a review of the effectiveness of health promotion interventions?

Table 3.2 *An example of a hierarchy of evidence (source: NHS CRD, 1996b). Reproduced with permission*

I	Well-designed randomized controlled trials
	Other types of trial:
II–1a	Well-designed controlled trial with pseudo-randomization
II–1b	Well-designed controlled trials with no randomization
	Cohort studies:
II–2a	Well-designed cohort (prospective study) with concurrent controls
II–2b	Well-designed cohort (prospective study) with historical controls
II–2c	Well-designed cohort (retrospective study) with concurrent controls
II-3	Well-designed case-control (retrospective) study
III	Large differences from comparisons between times and/or places with and without intervention. (In some circumstances these may be equivalent to level II or I)
IV	Opinions of respected authorities based on clinical experience; descriptive studies and reports of expert committees

experimental or quasi-experimental study), it is also true that all research needs to consider criteria of methodological validity. Consensus methods have been described which seek to synthesize information derived from qualitative or "grey" (unpublished) sources. These methods use laypeople or experts to assess information (Jones and Hunter, 1995). Ways forward are to encourage and facilitate greater collaboration and liaison between researchers and practitioners, and to enhance the research skills of practitioners (see Chapter 2 for more discussion about this issue).

In these studies it is the positivist framework of scientific research which determines the acceptability of evidence. Determining what should be measured to decide effectiveness depends on the objectives of the health promotion intervention and the particular model of health promotion being used. Traditionally this has been focused on the measurement of outcomes. Where it is difficult to demonstrate direct outcomes, intermediate and indirect indicators are used. The choice of indicators will depend on the objectives of the activity. Table 3.3 shows the range of indicators that could be used to evaluate oral health promotion for young people. In this case identifiable changes in individual behaviour are relatively easy to measure.

As we will see in the next section, focusing on behavioural outcomes is not appropriate for many health promotion activities such as community development work or working for policy change. In these cases, it is still possible to break down the objectives into specific indicators of effectiveness. What constitutes effective practice depends on what you choose to measure and this depends on your model and approach to health promotion.

What to measure

Five different models of health promotion – medical, educational, behavioural or lifestyles, social, and empowerment – will be examined in terms of the implications for evaluating the effectiveness of health promotion.

1. The medical model

The medical model of health promotion remains popular, as may be seen in the common assertion that the effectiveness of health promotion should be measured by its impact on preventing disease and increasing life expectancy (Reid, 1995).

D

A randomized controlled trial (RCT) is suggested to investigate the effect of an "exercise on prescription" scheme, whereby appropriate patients are referred to leisure centres to undertake subsidized and supervised exercise. The study would require eligible patients to be randomly allocated to either the "exercise on prescription" intervention group or to a control group. Both groups of patients would need to have their health status assessed pre- and post-intervention. What are the benefits and the problems of the proposed RCT?

The "gold standard" of medical effectiveness is the randomized controlled trial (RCT) which is described in Chapter 2. Using RCTs enables practitioners to be confident that a factor ("exercise on prescription" scheme) is or is not related to a specific outcome (improved health status).

However there are several problems with attempting to use RCTs in health promotion, the most obvious being timescale. If health promotion is effective in reducing risk factors for disease (e.g. reduction in smoking rates; increased rates of physical activity; adoption of healthier diets), the time-lag between these changes and final

Table 3.3 *Indicators to evaluate an oral health promotion programme for young people*

Outcome indicators	
Health status	Incidence of decay
	Incidence of peridontal disease
Behavioural measures	Reported dental hygiene measures (flossing, brushing)
	Reported reduction in sugar intake and frequency of sugar intake
Knowledge and attitude measures	Knowledge of correct brushing
	Knowledge of links between sugar and decay
	Positive attitudes towards dental hygiene practices
Self-concept measures	Values and beliefs about appearance
	Measures of self-esteem
Intermediate indicators	
Output indicators	Number of clients seen
	Number of materials distributed
Input indicators	Human and financial resources given to programme
Social policy indicators	Reduction in advertising of confectionery
	Reduction in availability of confectionery (e.g. in supermarkets, school tuck shops)
Process indicators	Number of organizations/agencies involved, e.g. in healthy alliances
	Oral health policy development and implementation

outcomes in terms of reduced morbidity and premature death is a matter of years, even decades. It is often impractical and costly to set up a five, ten or fifteen year research project to carry out a long-term evaluation of health promotion. Even if such a research project was established, it would be impossible to claim reduced morbidity and mortality resulted from particular interventions carried out years before. On-going activities and changes in lifestyles, social conditions and healthcare provision and treatment would confound the attempt to ascribe cause to effect.

D

Some studies attempt to control for confounding factors or variables which may affect the outcome. For example, Moser *et al.* (1986) in a longitudinal study of the effects of unemployment on health found unemployment was associated with increased ill-health. The study controlled for social class (which is known to be associated with ill-health).
What other variables might have contributed to this outcome?

There are also practical and ethical problems in denying control populations certain activities which are likely to be effective in order to have a rigorous research design. Once services are provided for some groups, it is likely that demand for such services will grow, making it difficult to deny or withdraw services even if they are shown to be ineffective. For example, pregnant women now expect an ultrasound scan at some stage of their pregnancy, although there continues to be debate about the usefulness and possible side-effects of routine ultrasound scanning.

This problem is not unique to health promotion. It has been estimated that less than 20% of clinical interventions are based on scientifically acceptable evidence (e.g. of proven effectiveness through the use of RCTs) (Learmonth, 1996). For example, three of the top ten operations performed in the NHS – tonsillectomy, dilation and curettage and grommet insertion for glue ear – are of questionable effectiveness and efficiency (Appleby, 1995).

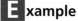**xample**

Stevens and Raftery (1994) cite the following activities which are of demonstrable effectiveness:

Salt reduction.
Smoking cessation.
Promotion of breast feeding.
CHD prevention programmes.
Immunization and vaccination programmes.
Accident reduction programmes.
Family planning, abortion and fertility services.
Screening for colorectal cancer.

The Health Care Evaluation Unit at the University of Bristol has investigated suicide and skin cancer prevention strategies (amongst others) and has identified effective health promotion strategies which merit immediate implementation (Gunnell, 1994; Harvey, 1995). Interestingly, this does not yet include a general population screening programme for skin cancer or the maintenance of anti-depressant and lithium therapy to prevent suicide, but does include primary health education measures about reducing skin exposure to the sun and sunbeds and the identification and environmental modification of local suicide "hotspots".

The best available evidence therefore supports the effectiveness of a variety of health promotion strategies as a means of preventing avoidable ill-health and death. However, there are specific problems with the evaluation of health promotion using RCTs, primarily the timescale, feasibility, and ethical implications.

A commonly proposed solution to these problems is to measure process or intermediate indicators that are markers for the desired long-term outcomes. In the example above, the take-up rate of immunizations and colorectal cancer screening are indicators of effectiveness because there is sound evidence that such activities reduce the burden of ill-health and premature death.

There is a growing body of research which enables practitioners to assess the long-term effects of interventions by extrapolating the effects of changes in indicators on longer-term outcomes. For example, the recent British Family Heart Study (1994) measured the reduction in cardiovascular risk factors achieved by screening and lifestyle advice. Lifestyle changes were used to estimate the reduction in heart attacks if they were maintained. This study concludes that an average reduction in risk factors of 12% would lead to a 1–2% reduction in mortality over one year. It is then necessary to decide whether such evidence makes this type of intervention effective. One means of doing this is to assess its cost-effectiveness. The concept of cost-effectiveness is discussed on p. 61.

Another intermediate indicator is the take-up of services which might be assumed to lead to a reduction in mortality and morbidity. Service utilization is relatively easy to measure. Many indicators of service use are already routinely collected and may be used by managers to assess the effectiveness of health promotion activities.

D

What intermediate indicators could you use to assess the effectiveness of the service you provide?
Are these indicators already available? If not, can you realistically measure them?
How strong is the research evidence linking service take-up with health outcomes?

2. The educational model

The educational model of health promotion seeks to provide advice and information to enable informed decisions. It is a well established and valued strategy. Attempts to examine effectiveness and the impact of educational interventions on health-related outcomes are relatively straightforward. Target populations may be divided into experimental groups which receive educational inputs and control groups, which do not. Pre- and post-testing of knowledge and skills is feasible. The size and nature of non-respondents or drop outs may be noted and commented on. A recent review of sexual health education interventions for young people found, however, that most interventions are not evaluated. Of those that are, few studies reached the minimum criteria of methodological soundness (Oakley *et al.*, 1995). Many studies report the process of educational interventions and the experience of participants but few explore the effect of the intervention on changing behaviour.

D Is an evaluation in terms of changes in behaviour appropriate for an educational intervention?

A large review of school-based health education programmes concluded that they "... consistently improve targeted health knowledge, attitudes and skills and inconsistently improve target health behaviours" (Tones and Tilford, 1994:145). An evaluation of drug education in Scotland (Coggans *et al.*, 1991), for example, found that drug education had an effect on drug-related knowledge but not on other outcome measures including drug-related perceptions and attitudes and pupils' self-reported drug use. Oakley and colleagues (1995) found that many studies which look at the effects of sex education do not even examine behavioural outcomes and only look at increases in knowledge. Of those studies which were methodologically sound, only two showed short-term effects on young people's reported sexual behaviour.

Tones and Tilford (1994) state that the quality of the planning process is the best predictor for effectiveness. The quality of the planning process may be assessed by using the following criteria:

- *Relevance* – that the intervention is relevant to the needs of the target audience.
- *Individualization* – that the intervention is targeted towards individual circumstances.
- *Feedback* – that feedback is given to the learner about any achievements.
- *Reinforcement* – that different media and means are used to reinforce the message.
- *Facilitation* – that the intervention enables the learner to take action to reduce barriers to action.

Activity

Take a health education activity with which you are familiar. Using the planning criteria consider how you could improve the effectiveness of the activity.

Tones and Tilford (1994:163–64) state that there are many examples of success in enhancing knowledge and information through health education carried out in healthcare settings, but that evidence of effectiveness in encouraging preventive behaviour is sparse. Nevertheless they conclude that: "On the basis of existing knowledge if proven interventions were routinely applied across health care settings as a whole, significant gains could be achieved" (Tones and Tilford, 1994:176).

3. The behavioural or lifestyles model

Behaviour is the indicator which is most often measured in health promotion research. Measurements of behaviour tend to treat it as an individually chosen attribute. For example, smoking is usually considered to be a freely chosen individual behaviour. Yet we also know that social class, income, gender and ethnicity are significantly associated with the likelihood of smoking. Smoking behaviour is also affected by the environment, whether or not smoking is prohibited or allowed in particular contexts. Measuring changes in social or environmental factors known to be associated with smoking may be easier and as relevant as measuring the behaviour of individuals.

> "the fundamental aim of an educational campaign is not simply to alter individual behaviour, but to alter some of the basic threads of the social fabric"
>
> (WHO, cited in Reid, 1995).

The effectiveness of mass media campaigns in changing behaviour is disputed (see Chapter 6), but one recent review concludes that paid advertising campaigns have "generally been associated with favourable outcomes when used appropriately" (Reid, 1995:12). Positive outcomes include adoption of sun protection behaviour, physical activity, increased condom sales, and smoking cessation.

Recently there have been proposals to research behaviour in ways which take account of social and environmental factors which affect behavioural choices and outcomes (Poland, 1992; Duncan *et al.*, 1996).

D

The message to take moderate exercise three times a week will be influenced by a variety of factors e.g.

- Attitudes to exercise.
- Available time for exercise.
- Exercise facilities and opportunities.

- Safety aspects of exercise.
- Beliefs about personal ability to exercise.

Whilst these are factors affecting individuals, they are also patterned by social and environmental aspects e.g. gender, social class, ethnicity, organizational policies, and leisure facilities. Enabling a group of Asian women (who may have less personal time due to caring responsibilities and who may feel unsafe in public areas and uncomfortable in general facilities) to take regular exercise may be more difficult and require greater inputs than enabling a group of single young men to exercise regularly.

Should these differences be reflected in the measurement of effectiveness? If so, how?

Both the use of qualitative methodologies (Poland, 1992) and the extension of quantitative methodologies to take account of contextual aspects (Duncan *et al.*, 1996) have been advocated as the way forward. The measurement of behavioural change is an important means of evaluating the effectiveness of health promotion but viewing behaviour solely as an individual variable does not do justice to the complexity of behavioural choices and change.

4. *The social model*

The social model of health promotion concerns the wider socio-economic environment as well as acknowledging that health is not just about prevention of disease and increased longevity, but is concerned with maximizing well-being. Well-being depends on many factors both internal and external; equity, participation, empowerment and a supportive social environment are all vital (WHO, 1986). It therefore follows that criteria for establishing the effectiveness of health promotion should include indicators of these factors as well as, or instead of, prevention of disease and longevity. A concern for equity for example would mean evaluating the accessibility of a health promotion intervention. Health education literature that is available only in English is an example of inequity given the multicultural and multilingual character of Britain. Equal access to services is an indicator of equality but not necessarily of equity.

D

Health screening clinics in primary health care settings are associated with changes in lifestyles and reductions in health risk behaviours. It is also known that such clinics are subject to the "inverse care law", whereby those most at risk make least use of such services (Pill *et al.*, 1988; Fowler and Mant, 1990; Waller *et al.*, 1990; Gillam, 1992; Davis *et al.*, 1996). Therefore, providing more health screening clinics may be effective (for users), yet at the same time contribute to health inequalities. Would you advocate more health screening clinics, on the grounds of their proven effectiveness?

Or would you argue for an alternative use of resources, e.g. targeting the most disadvantaged patients, on the grounds of equity?

There is substantial evidence that social inequalities undermine health and that inequalities in Britain have been widening in recent years (Townsend *et al.*, 1988; Wilkinson, 1994, 1996; Benzeval *et al.*, 1995). Epidemiological work has mapped the differences in health between population groups (Ahmad, 1993). In the previous chapter we saw how increased attention has also been given to lay experience and the ways in which individual behaviour is influenced by social conditions (Graham, 1996). There are numerous initiatives which attempt to address inequalities by, for example, making services more accessible; by monitoring the effects of policies to improve housing or provide work or by increasing the take-up of benefits. The evaluation of these initiatives has been local and what is measurable is often an inadequate indicator of complex processes (Laughlin and Black, 1995).

Example

The NHS Centre for Reviews and Dissemination (CRD)

The NHS CRD Report 3 (1995) is a review of the effectiveness of health service interventions to reduce variations in health. The report concludes that certain characteristics are associated with successful interventions (although their presence does not guarantee effectiveness). These characteristics are:

- Systematic and intensive approaches to delivering effective interventions, e.g. use of multiple media, multiple settings;
- Improving the accessibility of services;
- Prompts to encourage the use of services;
- Mutifaceted strategies;
- Collaborative strategies involving different interest groups;
- Interventions which address the expressed or identified needs of the target population;
- Involvement of peers in the delivery of interventions.

The review focused on interventions which the NHS could undertake, either alone or in collaboration with other agencies. It states that whilst removal of barriers to accessing healthcare is important, this will not by itself be sufficient to prevent all avoidable variations in health.

Changes in the socio-economic environment will require action across many sectors. The extent of intersectoral collaboration can be taken as an indicator of likely change in public policy although, as we discuss in Chapter 8, the process of such alliances needs to be analysed as well as their outcomes. Policy change or legislation may involve the use of indicators such as a healthy catering policy as well as the effect on health of changes in the environment. Qualitative methodologies are necessary to examine processes, and the conditions for quantitative or quasi-experimental or experimental research will often be lacking. For example, legislation will make a controlled study impossible, as the entire population will be affected by changes in the law.

E xample

Seat belts

Media-based educational campaigns to encourage the use of seat belts were unable to increase the level of use much above 30%, even though a majority claimed to have a positive attitude towards seat belt use. Subsequent legislation led to a vast majority of drivers complying with the requirement to use seat belts. However, it has been stressed that such compliance was facilitated by the preceding educational campaign (Tones and Tilford, 1994).

The difficulties in evaluation should not be used to marginalize the importance or effectiveness of such strategies in promoting health.

5. The empowerment model

For many health promoters, empowerment at an individual and/or collective level is a central tenet of health promotion (Tones, 1995). Empowerment is a difficult concept to measure, involving subjective assessments of change in personal autonomy and self-esteem and the development of skills to achieve desired ends. Some outcomes may be measurable, such as enhanced social networking or the achievement of changes in policy or service provision. However, research into the effectiveness of an empowerment model of health education is unlikely to meet scientific standards of replicability and representativeness.

The NHS CRD Review (1995) discussed on p. 59 excluded community development projects for these reasons. However, it has been argued that community development is too important to ignore on the grounds that evaluating its effectiveness is problematic (Taket, 1994). Beattie's (1991) review of evaluations of community development projects identified numerous qualitative evaluations such as action research, process and participatory evaluation, historical reviews and pluralistic strategies, which use both quantitative and qualitative approaches. Whilst many health promoters subscribe to this view (Learmonth, 1996), key audiences such as NHS managers or clinical practitioners remain resistant to accepting the validity of "soft" research methodologies investigating effectiveness.

This remains a problematic issue for health promoters. A key strategy for promoting health will be marginalized unless evidence of a qualitative nature is admitted in the effectiveness debate. It is important therefore to extend the effectiveness debate to include indicators of health enhancing processes. These might include support for client autonomy and participation, the development of healthy alliances and inter-agency collaborative working for health. Chapter 12 on mental health promotion includes a checklist for health promoters to identify indicators of empowerment.

D

Health promotion in a rural community

A health promoter is concerned about the high rate of suicide in rural communities, but is keen for the villagers to identify their own health needs. The project continued for two years in which the villagers:

■ Lobbied for improvements in the local bus service (an extra midday bus was added to the timetable);

■ Won a grant to fund a minibus to provide transport for parents and children to the nearest leisure centre, local outings, etc.;

■ Set up a farmers' information and support group.

What criteria would you use to demonstrate the effectiveness of the project in order to prolong its funding?

Cost-effectiveness

Increasing pressure on public spending in recent years has led to a concern to demonstrate the balance between costs and effectiveness. An effective intervention may be very high in human and financial resources and there may be other projects which are considerably cheaper and only slightly less effective. Cost-effectiveness analysis compares the costs of different interventions with the same aim (e.g. smoking cessation clinics compared with GPs prescribing nicotine replacement).

> "Cost-effectiveness analysis can be used either to identify the intervention which achieves a specific target at lowest cost or that which achieves the greatest outcome for a given cost"
>
> (Tolley, 1994:vii).

The analysis may include looking at opportunity costs – the value of using resources for health promotion rather than for alternative uses (alternative health promotion activities, treatment, other public spending programmes).

Where interventions differ in their success and in their costs, it becomes necessary not only to cost the intervention but also to put a price on the benefits resulting from the intervention. This leads to a calculation of the cost per given benefit (cost–benefit ratio). This enables a comparison to be made between interventions and also assesses whether an intervention is worthwhile in terms of the savings which might result (e.g. costs of routine nicotine replacement versus the financial benefits of smoking cessation).

D What problems can you identify in the use of cost-effectiveness analysis applied to health promotion?

Economic evaluation requires a rigorous study design, which is best achieved through experimental or quasi-experimental interventions. (see pp. 53–54 for problems posed). Economic evaluation relies on appropriate outcome measures – process indicators, intermediate outcomes or final outcomes. Final outcomes are, as we have seen, difficult to study because of timescale. Health promotion benefits tend to be long-term and therefore less persuasive than measures demonstrating immediate benefits. It is axiomatic in economic evaluation that people prefer to delay costs but reap immediate benefits.

> "Health education is generally more cost-effective than health care in the long term, but is likely to be less popular because its benefits are so difficult to demonstrate"
>
> (Reid, 1995:14).

Tones and Tilford (1994) caution against the wholesale adoption of cost-effectiveness criteria on the grounds that health represents a moral good (which cannot be costed) and because health promotion may in the long term lead to increased costs rather than savings (increased longevity is associated with increased costs via pensions and health and welfare services).

Nevertheless, economic evaluation of cost-effectiveness is a powerful means of establishing the validity of health promotion. Although still in its infancy, results are promising. Reid (1995) cites brief advice from a GP and participation in No Smoking Day as the two most cost-effective smoking cessation interventions.

Example

Smoking cessation strategies

The UK National No-Smoking Day is estimated to achieve a permanent quit rate of 0.5% of all adult smokers or 50,000 people per annum at an approximate annual cost of £1 million. This produces an estimated cost of £20 per quitter. A national mass media campaign is estimated to result in 750,000 quitters after a few months (assuming a higher quit rate of 5%); producing a cost per quitter of approximately £13. (Reid *et al.*, 1992.)

D

Reid *et al.* (1992) cite evidence from the USA that workplace health promotion interventions result in savings to employers of at least three times the cost.
What factors might be used to establish costs and benefits in this case?

The costs of workplace health promotion programmes include staff time and resources. Benefits are factors such as an enhanced corporate image and reductions in absenteeism, sick leave and staff turnover (leading to reductions in the cost of recruitment and training of staff) which save money and increase productivity. In the USA, a successful programme leading to a reduction in the cost of health insurance cover for companies is also counted as an economic benefit (Reid *et al.*, 1992).

It is apparent that what is measured in terms of effectiveness depends on what objectives are set for health promotion. The scientific paradigm centred on the experimental method is often inappropriate for health promotion, which is concerned with long-term outcomes, processes and indicators. Health promotion uses multiple evaluation strategies incorporating a variety of indicators. This in turn means there are many different audiences with different agendas who take an interest in the effectiveness of health promotion – practitioners, funders and researchers, as well as clients.

Who is the audience?

The effectiveness debate has been stimulated by recent NHS reforms which emphasize value for money and proven effectiveness of interventions. Yet the audience for research into effectiveness is broader. Professional colleagues, the public who are the focus of health promotion activities, employers and managers all constitute a potential audience. The intended audience of effeeveness research will impact on the kinds of strategies used. To date, the debate has been confined to professionals and policy makers, via professional journals and bodies conducting reviews of practice. It is argued that peer review is necessary in order to ensure high standards and the use of scientific criteria. There is, however, a contrary point of view, that the debate should extend to involve the public. Accountability is not just to employers, managers, funders or peers. The public pay for health promotion (through taxation) and have the right to be involved in appraising effectiveness. The health promotion principle of participation is not confined to implementation of strategies; it includes participation in appropriate research to determine effectiveness.

R ■ Do you use client/user feedback to appraise your health promotion activities?
■ Is it feasible to do this? Useful?
■ What problems can you foresee?

A second point follows on from this multiplicity of audiences. Audiences vary in the criteria they adopt, the kinds of evidence they find persuasive and what is seen as the purpose of health promotion. In order to meet the needs of different audiences, multiple research strategies are required. There is no one way of assessing effectiveness. Different research methodologies each have a role to play. Whilst each interest group may have its preferred means of assessing effectiveness (e.g. the randomized controlled trial for medical practitioners), greater efforts to communicate across occupational or social boundaries can be expected to have positive results in terms of clarifying goals and outcomes, prioritizing these, and refining research strategies.

Conclusion

It is important to be clear about the limits of evaluating effectiveness, and a necessary first step is to link the measurement of effectiveness to a theory of what health promotion aims to achieve and the processes involved in achieving these aims. This gives rise to a number of competing models of health promotion. It is significant that positive evaluations of the impact of health promotion have been reported for all these models (as well as failures or ineffectual interventions). Advances in health promotion depend upon wider recognition of the benefits resulting from the varied forms of health promotion activities, and more detailed investigations of what characteristics and factors are associated with success.

Taking an overview of health promotion, it is evident that no one method of practice or evaluation is the best for all situations. The experimental design which seeks to establish cause and effect is not appropriate for all interventions. Indicators that relate to process are as important. Health promoters should seek to resist medical dominance by asserting the validity of qualitative evaluation of processes as well as quantitative evaluation of outcomes. A prerequisite for this to happen is increased and improved communication between practitioners and researchers. The dissemination of findings, negative as well as positive, is often neglected – more should be done to open up the debate around effectiveness with a variety of audiences. Effectiveness and evidence-based practice is now on the agenda of health promoters, but often at the behest of medical or managerial personnel. Health promoters should seek to become more proactive in setting the terms of the debate and in becoming involved in the measurement of success.

Recommended reading

- HEA (1995) *Health Promotion Today*, London, Health Education Authority.
  Three articles examine the effectiveness of health promotion strategies including the use of the mass media, local and national strategies and empowerment strategies.

- The Health Care Evaluation Unit, University of Bristol.
  A series of recent reports evaluating different strategies. Topics reported on include skin cancer, suicide, antenatal care and pre-conception care. The reports are literature reviews and categorize interventions in terms of three levels; I (immediate implementation justified), D (monitored development justified to assess implementation) and R (evaluation research necessary to assess the implications of implementation).

- The NHS Centre for Reviews and Dissemination at the University of York.
  A series of reports and newsletters (*Effectiveness Matters* and *Effective Health Care Bulletin*) which aim to disseminate evidence of effectiveness provided by good research.

- Tones K and Tilford S (1994) *Health education: Effectiveness, efficiency and equity*, 2nd edn, London, Chapman and Hall.
  This comprehensive book gives details of numerous studies investigating the effectiveness of health promotion activities in different settings as well as providing a framework for considering the major issues involved.

- Hawe P, Degeling D and Hall J (1993) *Evaluating health promotion: A health worker's guide*, London, Maclennan and Petty.
  A practical guide to evaluation which considers the skills needed at different stages in the evaluation process. A useful glossary and annotated bibliography are included.

- Tolley K (1994) *Health promotion: How to measure cost-effectiveness*, London, Health Education Authority.
  A discussion of the issues involved in assessing cost-effectiveness.

References

Ahmad WIU (ed.) (1993) *"Race" and health in contemporary Britain*, Buckingham, Open University Press.

Appleby J (1995) The top ten 1995, *Health Service Journal*, 9/3/95.

Bachmann M and Nelson S (1996) *Screening for diabetic retinopathy: A quantitative overview of the evidence, applied to the populations of Health Authorities and Boards*, Bristol, Health Care Evaluation Unit, University of Bristol.

Beattie A (1991) "The evaluation of community development initiatives in health promotion: A review", in *Roots and branches, Papers from the OU/HEA 1990 Winter School on Community Development and Health*. Milton Keynes, Health Education Unit, Department of Community Education, Open University.

Benzeval M, Judge K and Whitehead M (1995) *Tackling inequalities in health: an agenda for action*, London, King's Fund.

Bredow M and Harvey I (1995) *Screening for fragile X syndrome*, Bristol, Health Care Evaluation Unit, University of Bristol.

British Family Heart Study (1994) "Randomised control trial evaluating cardiovascular screening and intervention in general practice: principal results of the British Family Heart Study", *British Medical Journal*, **308,** 313–320.

Coggans N, Shewan D, Henderson M and Davies JB (1991) *National Evaluation of Drug Education in Scotland*, London, Institute for the Study of Drug Dependence, Research Monograph 4.

Davis BS, McWhirter MF and Gordon DS (1996) "Where needs and demands diverge: health promotion in primary care", *Public Health*, **110,** 95–101.

Duncan C, Jones K and Moon G (1996) "Health-related behaviour in context: A multilevel modelling approach", *Social Science and Medicine*, **42,** 817–30.

Eiser JR and Eiser C (1996) *Effectiveness of Video for Health Education: A Review*, London, HEA.

Fowler G and Mant D (1990) "Health checks for adults", *British Medical Journal*, **300,** 1318–20.

Gillam SJ (1992) "Provision of health promotion clinics in relation to population need: another example of the inverse care law?", *British Journal of General Practice*, **42,** 54–56.

Graham H (1996) "Research on women and poverty: trends and future directions", in Daykin N and Lloyd L (eds) *Researching women, gender and health: Report of a conference held at the University of the West of England 17 June 1995*, Bristol, Faculty of Health and Social Care, University of the West of England.

Gunnell D (1994) *The potential for preventing suicide: A review of the literature on the effectiveness of interventions aimed at preventing suicide*, Bristol, Health Care Evaluation Unit, University of Bristol.

Harvey I (1995) *Prevention of skin cancer: A review of available strategies*, Bristol, Health Care Evaluation Unit, University of Bristol.

Health Care Evaluation Unit (1996) *Diagnosis, management and screening of early localised prostate cancer: a systematic review*, Bristol, Health Care Evaluation Unit, University of Bristol.

HEA (1993a) *Giving up Smoking: Does Patient Education Work?* London, Health Education Authority.

HEA (1993b) *Nutrition Interventions in Primary Health Care: A Literature Review*, London, Health Education Authority.

HEA (1996a) *Health Promotion in Children and Young Adolescents for the Prevention of Unintentional Injuries*, London, Health Education Authority.

HEA (1996b) *Health Promotion in Older People for the Prevention of Coronary Heart Disease and Stroke*, London, Health Education Authority.

HEA (1996c) *Health Promotion and Young People*, London, Health Education Authority.

HEA (1997a) *Health Promotion with Young People for the Prevention of Alcohol Misuse*, London, Health Education Authority.

HEA (1997b) *Health Promotion with Young People for the Prevention of Substance Misuse*, London, Health Education Authority.

Jones J and Hunter D (1995) "Consensus methods for medical and health services research", *British Medical Journal*, **311,** 376–80.

Laughlin S and Black D (1995) *Poverty and health: Tools for change*, Birmingham, Public Health Alliance.

Learmonth A (1996) *Society of Health Education and Promotion Specialists Position Paper on Health Gain, Effectiveness and Health Promotion: Draft*, SHEPS. (SHEPS is a professional society – at present, correspondence address is c/o North Cumbria Health Authority, Carlisle, Cumbria, CA1 1PT.)

Moody D, Aggleton P, Kapila M, Pye M and Young A (1991) *Monitoring and Evaluating Local HIV/AIDS Health Promotion: A Review of Theory and Practice*, London, HEA.

Moser KA, Fox AJ and Jones DR (1986) "Unemployment and mortality in the OPCS Longitudinal Study", in Wilkinson RG (ed.) *Class and health: Research and longitudinal data*, London, Tavistock.

NHS Centre for Reviews and Dissemination (1995) *Review of the Research on the Effectiveness of Health Service Interventions to Reduce Variations in Health*, CRD Report 3, York, University of York/NHS CRD.

NHS Centre for Reviews and Dissemination (1996a) *Ethnicity and Health: Reviews of Literature and Guidance for Purchasers in the Areas of Cardiovascular Disease, Mental Health and Haemoglobinopathies*, York, University of York/NHS CRD.

NHS Centre for Reviews and Dissemination (1996b) *Undertaking Systematic Reviews of Research on Effectiveness: CRD Guidelines for those Carrying Out or Commissioning Reviews*, CRD Report 4, York, University of York/NHS CRD.

Oakley A, Fullerton D, Holland J, Arnold S, France-Dawson M, Kelley P and McGrellis S (1995) "Sexual health education interventions for young people: a methodological review", *British Medical Journal*, **310,** 158-62.

Pearson V (1993) *Screening for Ovarian Cancer*, Bristol, Health Care Evaluation Unit, University of Bristol.

Pearson V (1994a) *Antenatal ultrasound screening*, Bristol, Health Care Evaluation Unit, University of Bristol.

Pearson V (1994b) *Preconception care*, Bristol, Health Care Evaluation Unit, University of Bristol.

Pearson V (1994c) *Frequency and timing of antenatal visits*, Bristol, Health Care Evaluation Unit, University of Bristol.

Pearson V (1995) *Antenatal genetic screening*, Bristol, Health Care Evaluation Unit, University of Bristol.

Pill R, French J, Harding K and Stott N (1988) "Invitation to attend a health check in a general practice setting: comparison of attenders and non-attenders", *Journal of the Royal College of General Practitioners*, **38,** 53–56.

Poland BD (1992) "Learning to 'walk our talk': the implications of sociological theory for research methodologies in health promotion", *Canadian Journal of Public Health*, **83,** 31.

Reid D (1995) "Is health education effective?", in *Health Promotion Today*, London, Health Education Council.

Reid D, Killoran A, McNeill A and Chambers J (1992) "Choosing the most effective health promotion options for reducing a nation's smoking prevalence", *Tobacco Control*, **1,** 185–97.

Richards SH (1995) *Prenatal Diagnosis: Amniocentesis or Chorion Villus Sampling*, Bristol, Health Care Evaluation Unit, University of Bristol.

Sprod A, Anderson R and Treasure E (1996) *Effective Oral Health Promotion: A Literature Review*, Cardiff, Health Promotion Wales.

Stevens A and Raftery J (eds) (1994) *Health Care Needs Assessment*, Oxford, Radcliffe Medical Press.

Taket A (1994) *Methodological Issues in the Evaluation of Health Promotion and their Relevance to the Modelling of Noncommunicable Diseases*. Paper given at a meeting organized by WHO and the Heidelberg Academy of Sciences, Heidelberg, September 1994.

Tolley K (1994) *Health promotion: How to Measure Cost-effectiveness*, London, Health Education Authority.

Tones K (1995) "Health education as empowerment", in *Health Promotion Today*, London, Health Education Authority.

Tones K and Tilford S (1994) *Health Education: Effectiveness, Efficiency and Equity*, 2nd edn, London, Chapman and Hall.

Townsend P, Davidson N and Whitehead M (1988) *Inequalities in Health: The Black Report and the Health Divide*, London, Penguin.

Waller D, Agass M, Mant D, Coulter A, Fuller A and Jones L (1990) "Health checks in general practice: another example of inverse care?", *British Medical Journal*, **300,** 1115–18.

Wilkinson RG (1994) *Unfair shares: The effects of widening income differences on the welfare of the young*, London, Barnardos.

Wilkinson RG (1996) *Unhealthy societies: The afflictions of inequality*, London, Routledge.

World Health Organization (1986) "Ottawa Charter for health promotion", *Journal of Health Promotion*, **1,** 1–4.

Dilemmas in Practice

Introduction

In 1987 the member states of the World Health Organization formulated a Global Strategy to disseminate existing Health For All principles. The strategy emphasized the complex nature of health and that action must take place at individual, community and structural levels. The strategy committed member states to the following principles:

- a holistic view of health;
- recognition of the environmental determinants of health;
- reducing inequalities in health;
- encouraging community participation;
- fostering intersectoral collaboration.

The Ottawa Charter for Health Promotion in 1986 incorporated the Health For All philosophy into health promotion policy which called for health promotion to:

- create supportive environments;
- enable community participation;
- develop personal skills for health;
- reorient healthcare services towards prevention and health promotion;
- build wide-ranging public policy which protects the environment and promotes health.

Part Two of this book looks at the dilemmas and challenges which arise when trying to put these principles into practice. Chapter 4 looks at the concept of equity and what this means for health promotion. Is it sufficient to work towards equal access to services or should health promotion attempt to reduce the inequalities in health between different groups? As poverty has been shown to be the principal determinant of health status, how is it possible to promote health amongst poor people living in disadvantaged environments? Chapter 5 takes a central tenet of health promotion – targeting – and looks at the assumptions and beliefs which underpin the belief that equity and effectiveness are achieved through prioritizing groups or health behaviours.

Chapter 6 takes the theme of marketing and looks at how marketing principles are being widely adopted in health promotion to put across health messages. It explores the assumptions of such an approach and questions whether marketing health may reinforce inequalities. Chapter 7 looks at the values and beliefs which underpin attempts to reorient health towards primary care and how this affects the practice of health promotion. Finally in this section, Chapter 8 looks at intersectoral collaboration and how this relates to the WHO principle of building a healthy public policy. It looks at the emphasis in the NHS on "healthy alliances" and the opportunities and constraints this offers for health promotion.

4 Promoting equity in health promotion: health and poverty

Key points

- Definitions of equity.
- Definitions of poverty.
- The link between poverty and ill-health.
- Barriers to promoting health in poverty.
- Strategies for promoting health in poverty.

Overview

Equity is a key principle in health promotion, endorsed by the World Health Organization in its Ottawa Charter (WHO, 1986). But what exactly does equity mean in health promotion, and how can health promoters seek to encourage equity in their practice? There are different definitions of equity, ranging from equal access to broad social reforms which seek to reduce social inequalities. Evidence has been collected on the differences in health status and health-related behaviours across social groups, e.g. those relating to social class, gender and ethnicity (Benzeval *et al.,* 1995; Doyal, 1995; Smaje, 1995). What the Department of Health called "social variations" remain wide (DoH, 1995). One of the main causes of inequalities is poverty and this chapter focuses on the inequalities in health which are associated with poverty.

The chapter first looks at definitions of equity and poverty and examines the evidence for poverty as a feature of modern British life. It then goes on to give a brief review of the research investigating the links between poverty and ill-health. The response to poverty at different levels (social, organizational and individual) is discussed. Examples of projects which seek in different ways to promote health amongst low income clients in deprived areas are given and questions raised by these examples are discussed.

Defining equity

Equity, or being fair and just, is not the same as equality, which is the state of being equal. It is unrealistic to expect we can ever attain equality in health, but it is important that in health, as in other areas, decisions and their effects seek to provide fair and just services and outcomes.

R ■ How would you define equity in health?
■ In what ways do you or could you promote equity in your work?

Some people argue that equity means equality of access to appropriate services, which is achieved through providing the same services for everyone. However, if people have different needs, then providing a universal service will not necessarily meet these differing needs fairly. People who face specific barriers in accessing services (e.g. homeless people, those whose first language is not English, carers who find it difficult to make time to meet their own needs) may need additional or specific provision in order to be able to access services. This chapter is not about equality of access to services. Other chapters discuss these issues; for example, Chapter 7 on primary healthcare notes the ways in which healthcare reforms may increase inequalities and how services which are not targeted to reducing inequalities in access (e.g. screening) are unlikely to be successful.

Others argue that equity means working to reduce inequalities in health. Research shows inequalities in health still exist, and that the major cause of such inequalities is poverty (Benzeval *et al.,* 1995). Poverty is a controversial issue and the next section explores definitions and meanings further. Practitioners may seek to promote the health of people living in poverty through specific strategies such as targeting or the development of community activities. Or they may argue that the key task is to ensure that no one lives below the poverty line, and that there is a general redistributive shift in incomes in order to narrow the gap between the rich and the poor. These broad-ranging changes can only be achieved through welfare and social policies focusing on issues such as redistributive taxation, minimum wages and adequate benefit levels. Local initiatives can also make an impact by, for example, ensuring that people receive their full benefit entitlement (see pages 82–83 for a discussion of such a project).

Defining poverty

At the heart of much of the debate around inequalities in health is a debate concerning poverty – what it is and how it should be defined.

R ■ How would you define poverty?
■ Is poverty different to inequality? How?

In the Reflection point, did you define poverty in terms of:

■ not having enough to eat or not having access to adequate housing (absolute poverty);
■ not having the minimum necessary to take part in social activities or afford a lifestyle commonly regarded as appropriate and desirable (relative poverty).

Poverty may be defined as absolute poverty – the inability to meet basic biological needs such as food, warmth and shelter. The welfare system is designed to act as a safety net, ensuring that no one falls through into absolute want or destitution. Using this definition, Conservative politicians claimed that poverty in the absolute sense of want was not an issue. Instead, they claimed that different cultures, lifestyles and health beliefs led to variations in health status, or inequality. Inequality was viewed as a positive attribute of society which rewarded the enterprising and provided incentives to produce more. The benefits of an unequal society "trickle down" to reach all strata of society (George and Wilding, 1994). The effect of policies predicated on this notion polarized the haves and have nots even further, resulting in wider discrepancies in income between the highest and lowest income groups (DSS, 1992).

Relative poverty means poverty defined in relation to the living standards and expectations of contemporary society.

D

Which of the following items do you consider necessary to provide an acceptable lifestyle and standard of living in the UK today, and which adults should be able to afford for themselves or their families?

- Washing machine
- Refrigerator
- Damp-free home
- Television
- Carpets in the home
- All-weather shoes and winter coat
- Money for children's birthday presents
- Video
- Car

(Mack and Lansley, 1985, report the results of a public opinion survey which included this question.)

Townsend (1979:31) defines relative poverty as

> "when (individuals) lack the resources to obtain the types of diet, participate in the activities and have the living conditions and amenities which are customary, or at least widely encouraged or approved, in the societies to which they belong."

D In what ways does poverty restrict people's lives?

Poverty is about exclusion, marginalization and the inability to participate in society as well as low income. Poor people are those who, because of their low income, are unable to participate in many of the activities which society regards as normal or appropriate. Social contacts are reduced, the pursuit of individual interests is likely to be impossible, and choices are severely constrained. In a sense, poor people become second class citizens, without the resources to enjoy what constitutes everyday life for most people.

It is possible therefore to have widespread relative poverty in societies which are wealthy. This is sometimes referred to as inequality, with the implication that inequality is not a significant problem. An unequal distribution of wealth is as significant as the total amount of wealth in analysing poverty. Recent research suggests that relative poverty, or the unequal distribution of social resources, is closely linked to health status (Wilkinson, 1993, 1996; Blane *et al.*, 1996). Affluent countries with unequally distributed resources have populations with poorer health status than countries with equal distribution of resources.

> "The results of a series of research projects . . . suggest that the degree of socio-economic inequality in developed countries is a key determinant of the *average* standard of health of their populations . . . among the rich developed countries, it is not the richest countries which have the highest life expectancy, but the ones with the most egalitarian distribution of income."
>
> (Wilkinson, 1993:7, original emphasis).

Conversely, poor countries with egalitarian resource distribution mechanisms and policies, such as Cuba, experience better than expected health status. Wealthy countries with redistributive policies, for example modern Japan, have the healthiest populations.

D Why do you think that it is not the richest countries that have the best health, but those that have the smallest income differences between rich and poor?

The close relationship between relative inequality and ill-health suggests that a crucial element is the psychological stress of experiencing poverty in an affluent society (Wilkinson, 1993, 1996). There is some evidence that stress is mediated through immunological and hormonal responses which may harm health (Madge and Marmot, 1987; House *et al.*, 1988). Poverty may also reduce the social support and social networks available to people, which have also been shown to be closely related to health (Brown and Harris, 1978; Cohen and Syme, 1985).

Measuring poverty

How to measure poverty has been the subject of much debate. Britain, unlike many other countries, does not have an official poverty line. Instead, most researchers and organizations use a measure of the percentage of the population subsisting on below average incomes. Two common measures are the percentage of the population subsisting on income support levels, or the percentage of the population subsisting on below 50% average income after housing costs (the European Union definition). Using these measures, the recent growth of poverty in Britain is well documented (Oppenheim, 1990).

Government sources show that, using a definition of poverty as the percentage of households with an income below 50% of the average, the number of people living in poverty increased from 4.9 million or 9% of the population in 1979, to 11.7 million or 22% of the population in 1988/9 (DSS, 1992). The poorest groups in society have not benefitted from the average increase in incomes (Figure 4.1). Between 1979 and 1987 average income increased by 23% whereas the poorest 10% of the population had an increase in income of just 0.1% (DSS, 1990, quoted in Blackburn, 1991). The share of income of the bottom fifth of households fell between 1981 and 1990/1, whilst only the top fifth had a larger share of total income in 1990/1 than they had in 1981 (Central Statistical Office, 1994).

D Which groups of people are more likely to be poor? Why?

The significant rise in relative poverty has been driven by low pay coupled with high unemployment rates. The following groups are therefore more likely to be poor:

- Low paid workers.
- Black or minority ethnic people.
- Disabled people.
- Women.
- Unemployed people.
- Households with children, especially lone parent households.
- Pensioners.

Discrimination in the labour market on the grounds of race, age, disability and gender leads to certain groups finding it more difficult to obtain secure employment (Glendinning, 1987; Harris, 1991; Amin and Oppenheim, 1992; Berthoud *et al.*, 1993). Low pay, defined as two thirds the average male wage, affected almost half of the workforce during the 1980s (Winyard and Pond, 1989). The greater vulnerability of certain groups to poverty is the outcome of a complex interaction of different factors, illustrated in the following example.

Figure 4.1 *The poverty gap in the UK this century.*

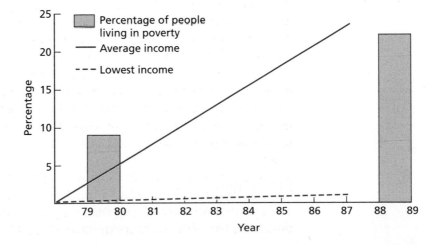

Women, especially lone parents (90% of whom are women; Blackburn, 1991:17) are likely to find themselves in the position of being low paid workers, mostly through working part time (Graham, 1993). Women with caring responsibilities who are unable to take a paid job may find themselves struggling to make do on inadequate benefits. It has also been recognized that within households with apparently adequate incomes, resources may be unevenly divided and so when there is a shortage it is women who do without (Graham, 1987b). Living on a low income has a particular significance for women, who have the responsibility and workload of caring within a context of reduced personal and material resources. For older women with less likelihood of a full entitlement to an occupational pension, there is an increased chance of poverty in old age. The term "feminization of poverty" has been coined to refer to this overall greater risk of poverty for women (Glendinning and Millar, 1992).

The lack of support for child care costs means that households with children, especially those headed by a lone parent, are more likely to be poor, as income is inadequate to pay for child care. The effect of this is that children are more likely than the rest of the population to be living in poverty. In 1987 when 19% of the population were poor, 26% of children were poor (Oppenheim, 1990:31). Families with dependent children now form the largest single group living in poverty, with 1 in 3 children currently living in poor households (Marsh and McKay, 1994).

There is a significant shortfall between benefit entitlement and take-up. The Department of Social Security estimated that in 1991 between 10% and 23% of those entitled to income support and 38% of those entitled to family credit did not claim their benefit (National Food Alliance, 1994). People who are entitled to benefit but do not claim it are amongst the poorest in society. Black people and people from ethnic minorities are least likely to receive their full benefit entitlement, due in part to racist attitudes or institutions (Blackburn, 1991). There is also the "poverty trap", whereby people may find themselves eligible for benefit but also paying tax. For some, any increase in earnings may lead to lost benefits and an overall worsening of their financial position. Taxation policies, such as the extension of Value Added Tax (VAT) to fuel, affect those on low income most. These regressive taxes take no account of income and are therefore a greater burden for poor people.

Explaining poverty

There are differing explanations for the persistence of poverty in a developed society. Some people see the poor as dependent on the state through laziness or indifference. George and Wilding (1994:31–34) discuss the view that welfare policies create dependency and undermine individual responsibility. Other people see poverty as the result of certain groups in society being excluded from economic and social life. Practitioners, who may work with poor clients or who may develop interventions to promote health amongst people with low incomes, need to think through their attitudes to poverty and the poor.

R

Consider the following newspaper headlines. How are poor people portrayed?

- Scrounger swindles tax payers of thousands in fraudulent benefits claims
- Claimants live it up on the Costa del Dole – at our expense!
- Aggressive beggars and squeegee merchants terrorize the streets
- Woman gets pregnant in order to get a council flat
- The lost children – lone parents' estate a ghetto of drink, drugs and prostitution

The first three headlines suggest a victim-blaming ideology which misconstrues people's circumstances as the cause of poverty, instead of recognizing that poverty is caused by much broader social policies. A victim-blaming ideology justifies the lack of a comprehensive anti-poverty strategy. Indeed, it has been argued that increased welfare benefit provision increases poverty through encouraging dependency. Such an ideology also perpetuates myths about the "deserving" and the "undeserving" poor. If poverty is attributed to different cultural norms, clients may be labelled as "deviants", encouraging judgemental attitudes towards their lifestyle and values. The fourth and fifth headlines indicate this kind of analysis.

Poverty and health – the evidence

That poverty is a major cause of ill-health and premature death is supported by the vast majority of academic and research studies, including those commissioned by the government (Townsend *et al.*, 1988; Shiell, 1991; Association of Community Health Councils, 1990; Wilkinson, 1989, 1993, 1994, 1996).

Poverty affects health in three main ways – physical, behavioural and psychological (Figure 4.2).

Example

Homelessness and health

Connelly and Crown (1994) found a clear relationship between homelessness and ill-health. They estimate that in 1991/2 there were:

- 169,966 families comprised of children or pregnant women who are the only group officially recognized as homeless;
- 2827 rough sleepers;

- 19,417 hostel dwellers;
- an unknown number of families sharing accommodation or inadequately housed.

Homelessness is caused by many different factors including family breakdown and domestic abuse, a shortfall in housing, especially of social-rented housing for low-income households, the government's "right to buy" policy and not enough new housing being built (Connelly and Crown, 1994). There are increased rates of physical and mental ill-health among homeless people. "This is probably related not only to their health problems but also to the difficulties they have in gaining access to primary care. For many of them, a 'healthy lifestyle' is unattainable in crowded accommodation with inadequate cooking and recreational facilities" (Connelly and Crown, 1994:xv).

D In what ways might homelessness or poor quality housing affect health?

Cold and damp housing gives rise to a variety of health problems including increased rates of:

- a variety of respiratory conditions including chronic bronchitis, asthma and emphysema;
- allergies;
- infections, e.g. tuberculosis and dysentery;
- accidental and violent deaths;

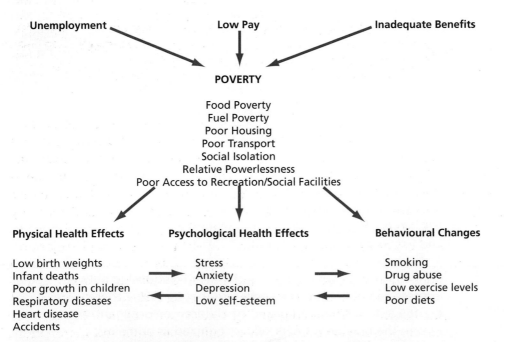

Figure 4.2   *How poverty affects health (Blackburn, 1992).*

- heart attack and stroke;
- cervical and lung cancer.

(Source: Standing Conference on Public Health, 1994)

Poor quality housing is difficult and expensive to heat. Excess mortality, from myocardial infarction, stroke and respiratory conditions, is linked to cold spells (Standing Conference on Public Health, 1994:31). The poor spend twice as much on heating (as a percentage of total income) as the rest of the population (Boardman, 1991). One study of families living on benefit found that 54% did not use their central heating as much as they wanted, 27% used central heating only very occasionally and a third never or rarely heated their bedrooms (Bradshaw and Holmes, 1989).

Poverty is more than the inability to meet basic physical needs. It is also about the inability to afford a standard of living which enables participation in everyday life (Townsend, 1979). It is about making do and being excluded from the choices which the better off take for granted including choices about diet and leisure activities.

R

- "Poor people bring illness upon themselves. They don't care about their health, they smoke and drink too much and eat junk food. They could spend the money on healthy activities if they really wanted."
- "The use of tobacco and alcohol, and the taking of both prescribed and unprescribed drugs . . . collectively referred to as 'drugs of solace' (Cameron and Jones, 1985), is often influenced by the quality of people's social relations and by factors such as stress and self-esteem" (Wilkinson, 1993:24).
- "(Smoking is seen as) providing a particularly important resource during the times of crisis that punctuate the lives of those struggling against material disadvantage" (Crossan and Amos, 1994:34).

Which of these three quotes comes closest to your view?

Research suggests that health risk behaviours should not be perceived as "wrong" lifestyle choices, but as rational coping strategies adopted in the context of the demands of caring and the constraints of poverty (Graham, 1987a). Graham (1996) argues that the transposition of epidemiological risk factors based on population studies to individually targeted advice and education is fundamentally flawed. Such a strategy fails to acknowledge the effects of poverty on people's own perceptions of health, risk and priorities. "Landscapes of risk" vary according to a person's social situation and status. Risk is relative, and priorities shift with changing circumstances (see Chapter 5 on targeting for a detailed discussion of this issue). Epidemiological risk factors such as smoking or poor diet may be overridden by more immediate risks and more urgent problems.

D   A key health promotion message is "Quit smoking". How will poverty affect how this message is received and interpreted?

A simplistic message such as "quit smoking" may refer to an avoidable risk for someone whose material needs are guaranteed and the health promotion message may be relevant and appropriate. On the other hand, smoking may be a necessary prop in order to cope with the immediate environment for someone living in poverty and the message may patronise, induce guilt or alienate such people. Smoking represents one of the . . .

> ". . . no-choice options for those struggling to make ends meet and make the best of caring in difficult circumstances"
>
> (Blackburn, 1993:299).

If this explanation for the known greater prevalence of smoking among poor people (Marsh and McKay, 1994) is accepted, it is unlikely that individually targeted information and advice on its own will have much impact on smoking behaviour.

A number of studies have shown that poor people eat less healthy diets than higher income people (HEA, 1989; Gregory *et al.*, 1990; NFA, 1994; Dowler and Calvert, 1995).

> "I see a good deal of old-fashioned low-intake malnutrition, especially among the long term unemployed; people who still survive on sweet tea, toast, chips and biscuits. Bread and margarine is a dietary staple in the 1990s as much as it was in the 1930s. Women commonly cut back on their food to feed their children and husband. Food is often short by the end of the week. In large families it often lacks variety, freshness and quality"
>
> (Widgery, 1993:113).

Whilst it is sometimes claimed that this is due to ignorance of nutrition messages, inefficient food purchasing or unwillingness to change, evidence suggests that poverty is the major barrier to improving diets. Chapter 9 on cardiovascular disease includes further discussion of nutrition interventions in health promotion.

Blackburn (1991, 1992) suggests that the failure to acknowledge the links between material conditions of people's lives and health has led to a situation where the bulk of health promotion programmes are targeted at individuals. In the examples of smoking and healthy eating above, we see how general health education messages are targeted to low income groups. Such strategies compound the exclusion and lack of control of low income groups by suggesting that individuals have a choice and responsibility for their health. The next section reviews the dilemmas and challenges that health promoters face in trying to promote health for those who are already disadvantaged. It discusses why there is such inaction on the links between poverty and health amongst health promoters themselves and at the level of public policy.

Barriers to effective health promotion in poverty

Since the publication of the Black Report (Townsend *et al.*, 1988) the relationship between income and health has been downplayed. Government inaction has represented the major barrier to promoting health in poverty. The new Labour government, however, is committed to reducing the extent and impact of poverty. The new Labour government's proposals to combat poverty include: a national minimum wage, using the income generated by the sale of council houses to build new homes, and getting young people into work.

Blackburn (1993) argues that the training of front line primary healthcare workers is a barrier to a coordinated anti-poverty strategy. Health promoters come from a variety of backgrounds and lack a common approach to poverty. The larger question about how theoretical knowledge and practice do and should interact has been discussed in more detail in Chapter 1.

Inadequate training is compounded by a lack of appropriate resources. Many resources provided for health promoters ignore the issue of poverty (DoH, 1993). By focusing on knowledge, attitudes or behaviour, the real constraints poverty imposes on healthy lifestyles are made invisible. Examples of resources which tackle the issue of poverty are Blackburn, 1992; Laughlin and Black, 1995; and Daykin *et al.*, 1995.

R ■ Think of a client or group of clients whom you would characterize as poor. What do you think are the causes of their poverty?
■ Do they see themselves as poor? If so, what do they see as the causes?
■ Are the two views the same?

For health promoters who recognize the effects of poverty, other barriers remain. Acknowledging the scale of the problem can lead to a feeling of helplessness (Blackburn, 1993). Healthcare professionals feel ill-equipped to address such problems, and relevant activities, for example supporting communal interventions such as food co-operatives, are often seen as falling beyond their remit. Such a situation can lead to low morale and frustration. This will be increased if the broader social policy arena is also perceived as unsupportive.

Promoting health in poverty: the response

Given the different kinds of barriers outlined above, it is clear that an adequate response would need to be made at many different levels. This section discusses three levels of response – the macro or social level, the meso or organizational level and the micro or individual level.

Macro level – an anti-poverty strategy
The complexity and many faceted nature of the relationship between poverty and ill-health suggests that it is not readily amenable to change via health promotion interventions. A genuine commitment

to tackling the inequalities in health resulting from poverty requires an integrated response at many different levels to produce a comprehensive anti-poverty strategy.

D What would you include in an anti-poverty programme?

The Black Report of 1980 (Townsend *et al.*, 1988) produced a blueprint for the kind of policies which would effectively promote health in poverty. As well as suggestions for more research and allocating resources according to need, the report called for a central body to co-ordinate policy to reduce inequalities in health, the abolition of child poverty through increased benefit levels, and an improved social housing programme. More recently, the King's Fund has produced a report of how to tackle inequalities in health (Benzeval *et al.*, 1995). This report identifies four factors which are amenable to change:

- the physical environment;
- social and economic influences;
- barriers to healthy lifestyles;
- access to appropriate and effective health and social services.

Suggestions for action to tackle these issues centre on government policies to increase income and access to the necessities for life, e.g. a minimum wage, employment policies that enable women to work (flexible hours, parental leave, affordable child care), increased income support and universal benefits, as well as the provision of appropriate and accessible services. George and Wilding (1994) show clearly how the New Right political ideology of the 1970s and 1980s was totally opposed to any purposeful collective enterprise which was seen as giving rise to a dependency culture.

The health strategy of the new Labour government, "Our Healthier Nation" (DoH, 1997) is committed to confronting the underlying causes of ill-health, reflecting their values of social justice. In July 1997, the Minister for Public Health, Tessa Jowell, described the challenge for the government as tackling the "persistent and damaging inequalities in health between different occupational and ethnic groups, between geographical areas and between men and women . . . Right across society, the poorer you are the less healthy you are likely to be" (DoH, 1997). The Labour Minister for Public Health recognized the need for a new analysis, which did not start from the premise that inequalities were an unavoidable fact of life and peripheral to healthy policy but which recognized the pervasive influences on health of social, economic and environmental policies.

Case study

Bristol Welfare Benefits Advice Service

This project, funded by the United Bristol Healthcare NHS Trust, provides an independent source of advice, information and advocacy on benefits for individual clients and health staff. It began life as a two-year pilot scheme under the auspices of the Bristol Inner City Health Project. Since then it has received funding from joint finance for two, three-year periods. Funding for 1990–1993 was approximately £25,000 per annum and for 1993–1996 approximately £57,000 per annum. The project's three welfare benefits advisers and administrative worker (all part time) operate from a Portakabin® based at an inner city health centre. An outreach service is provided to large outer city council estates. One adviser has a specific remit for homeless and travelling families. Clients may be referred, use the drop-in service, or be visited at home.

For each of the two years 1990/1 and 1991/2 over 2000 people received advice. The project also provided advocacy for clients and was involved in take-up campaigns to encourage full take-up of entitlements. The project estimates that the amount of benefit paid out as a result of the service's intervention was £500,000 for 1990/1 and £600,000 for 1991/2, an average of £4.76 per user. In practice, benefit entitlements vary enormously from one user to the next. But even a few pounds extra per week may "... make the difference between eating a healthy meal six days a week or every day of the week; to a pensioner it might mean the difference between risking hypothermia or having the heating on for a little longer each day" (Richards, 1990:20). In addition to this direct outcome, the project enables vulnerable people to remain in the community and frees health workers to deal with health problems. The service is also involved in local welfare rights forums and in the provision of specialist training (Richards, 1990, 1993).

How would you evaluate this project? What criteria would you use?

Compared to many other health promotion interventions, the welfare benefits advice service appears to be of proven effectiveness using a variety of criteria:

- The service avoids victim blaming by focusing on benefit entitlement not unhealthy lifestyles.
- Quantitative positive outcomes are apparent, both in terms of numbers of users, and in terms of additional income flowing into the area. The service has been used by many of the most marginalized groups, including homeless and travelling families.
- Qualitative outcomes are provided in the form of individual case studies where increased income leads to health benefits.
- The service is popular with health staff, who are able to refer clients to expert benefits advisors, leaving them free to concentrate on their area of expertise – health.

Other local initiatives are new models of savings, credit and exchange such as credit unions or local exchange trading schemes (LETS) which allow local trade by using credits instead of money. LETS are also intended to maximize employment opportunities by building up skills. Schemes which maximize or increase income, or provide services and stimulate trade via credits, provide the most direct example of tackling the links between poverty and health.

Meso level: organizational change

At the meso or organizational level, training and adequate resourcing should form part of an integrated response. Blackburn (1991) highlights the importance of practitioners providing a social commentary in their areas of the links between poverty and health. To do this, organizations need to recognize its importance and ensure that this is included in all community profiling and needs assessments. Strategies to ensure that all sections of the population have equal access to equal quality services might require the development of targeted healthcare provision. Dilemmas surrounding the issue of targeting are discussed in Chapter 5.

The professional training of many health workers, with its focus on the individual client, has been identified as a barrier to effective anti-poverty work (Blackburn, 1993). For many health promoters there is a strong professional ethos of one-to-one intervention which values and respects the individuality of each client. Factors common to people's health problems, such as poverty, tend to be overlooked. Blackburn's (1993) argument, that primary healthcare practitioners' training predisposes them to view poverty as posing additional burdens on health instead of being seen as the fundamental cause of much ill-health and premature death, has been referred to in Chapter 1. Blackburn found that practitioners consistently under-estimate the extent and impact of poverty on health, due in part to their own distance from poverty. This distance can lead to practitioners imposing advice or information which has little relevance to the lives of their clients.

R

- Has your training and education acknowledged the effect of poverty on health?
- What kind of analysis of poverty was given?
- What responses and strategies to tackle poverty have been discussed?
- What is your evaluation of the training and education which has been provided?

Community development work is often used to enhance quality of life and social support networks. For example, facilitating food co-operatives or "healthy food on a budget" sessions with local mothers might be more effective than repeating healthy food messages to women who know this information but are unable to act upon it. Getting people together to think about common problems may well have positive spin offs in terms of encouraging social support networks.

Example

The Wirral Women's Group

The Wirral Women's Group (WWG) was set up in the late 1980s by women in the local community to provide a means of networking, to support personal development and to lobby local authorities for accessible and appropriate services. Several years on, the Group has achieved many things. Women involved in the WWG have developed new skills and confidence, enabling them to take an active role in education, employment and voluntary agencies sectors. Together women have shared their experiences, recognized common problems and devised creative solutions. For example, a toy library and local transport were established in order to enable women to meet together. Changes in services provided e.g. outreach baby and well-women clinics and a local chemist, have been won through lobbying. The WWG has gone on to represent women's needs to local health, education and welfare authorities, as well as to national agencies such as the Health Education Authority (HEA video, 1991).

Community health projects may however be criticized for becoming insular. By focusing on local needs and services, the importance of challenging broader social organizations and structures may be missed (Laughlin and Black, 1995:66).

Researching local needs provides an opportunity to adopt a poverty perspective and to put into practice the principles of health promotion. Traditional needs assessment through epidemiological data is increasingly being supplemented with surveys of people's perceived priorities, conducted in a way which encourages participation (Blackburn, 1992; Laughlin and Black, 1995). Community profiling provides a basis for raising awareness, assessing needs and targeting services, and may be conducted at authority or more local levels. Individual primary healthcare practitioners, for example community nurses, may undertake such profiles for use as a planning and evaluation tool. Some practitioners may feel it is intrusive to ask people about their income. Explaining why you are asking this information and limiting the number of questions you ask are useful strategies. One simple question, "are you in receipt of income support?", will provide the necessary data to put poverty into community profiling.

D In what other ways could a poverty element be incorporated into needs assessments and the collection of information?

Micro level – the practitioner level

At the micro or individual level, training and resources to address poverty systematically and non-judgementally with clients need to be provided. In one-to-one health education work it is important that poverty is neither ignored (it is a central factor in determining health behaviour) nor seen as something individuals bring upon themselves.

Raising awareness of the issue is something which can be undertaken by individual practitioners, trainers, teachers and researchers.

A useful first step for all practitioners is to clarify ideas of what poverty is and how it affects clients, and how this is or is not acknowledged in everyday work. Understanding the structural causes of poverty and how it is mediated by factors such as age, disability, gender and race enables practitioners to avoid exacerbating problems by blaming people, explicitly or implicitly, for any unhealthy behaviours they may adopt. The way in which services are provided has an impact. Table 4.1 summarizes points for practice.

Practitioners may request or provide professional updates on poverty and health in order to have some protected time to think through the issues. There are some resource materials designed to assist this process (Blackburn, 1992; Daykin *et al.*, 1995; Laughlin and Black, 1995). In Chapter 1 we noted the importance of practitioners reflecting on their knowledge base and assumptions. This is particularly important in the case of poverty and health, which is an emotive issue impacting on the work of most practitioners.

Effective health promotion must include in its aims the reduction of inequalities in health which result from economic inequality. The most effective action is likely to be a broad shift in policy at the

Table 4.1 *Helpful and unhelpful health and welfare services*

Helpful	Unhelpful
An integrated approach	Services that treat financial, health and social problems as unrelated
A co-ordinated response	Individual agencies working on separate sets of problems
Services which offer realistic advice and recognise the limitations that poverty places on people	Providing help only when families are in crisis
	Interventions which individualise problems
Partnerships between families and workers where families' contributions are valued	Services based on what professionals think that families want rather than what families say they want
	Failure to recognise what families do achieve in adversity
	Blaming families for their poverty
Services that are permanent	Temporary or short term projects
Services that are relevant	Forcing families to define financial problems as emotional problems or personal inadequacy before help is given
Services that are easy to use	Only providing help when families are labelled as a problem

Reproduced from Laughlin and Black (1995), with permission

macro economic level. For practitioners this can be daunting and lead them to sidestep the issue of poverty as far beyond their remit. However there are a variety of ways in which health promoters, wherever they are located and whatever their role, can work towards reducing the unhealthy effects of inequality. The first step is to recognize the importance of equity as a guiding principle. For health promoters this means:

- social commentary – collecting data on how social and economic factors influence local health;
- accessible services – recognizing ways in which interventions and services can exclude those on low income;
- appropriate services – providing services which focus on client-defined issues and needs.

Conclusion

The link between poverty and ill-health is well known. There is strong evidence that, beyond a certain level of income (exceeded in all Western countries), what matters most is not absolute levels of income, but its relative distribution. Economic inequality is associated with increased ill-health amongst the poorer groups in society. This relationship is mediated by three mechanisms – physical, behavioural and psychological.

Many health promoters remain unconvinced by this analysis. Medical training and the individualized expert/client relationship downplays the importance of social and environmental factors in determining health status. Unhealthy behaviours may be attributed to ignorance or irresponsibility. Even if the relationship between poverty and health is acknowledged, health promoters may feel powerless to have any impact on the problem.

Case studies of a range of interventions designed to promote health in poverty indicate the variety of possible activities. An effective strategy to promote health requires interventions at different levels, from government policies on income distribution and employment through local policies on service provision and community development to individual contacts with clients. It is hoped that this chapter will encourage health promoters, wherever they are located, to identify the effects of poverty on health and to plan and implement strategies to address this problem. In the next chapter we look in detail at one strategy employed to address inequalities which is to target the most disadvantaged groups to ensure they have access to appropriate services.

Further discussion

- How could your health promoting role explicitly address inequalities?

- How would an understanding and analysis of social policy affect the type of health promotion interventions undertaken in your work?

- Complete the following questionnaire. What do your answers tell you about your understanding of, and attitudes towards, poverty?

	Agree	Don't know	Disagree
Poor people are victims of social forces beyond their control	☐	☐	☐
Poor people spend their money on luxuries they don't need	☐	☐	☐
Poor people envy those who have more money	☐	☐	☐
Poverty is a fact of life	☐	☐	☐
I am poor	☐	☐	☐
Poverty is inevitable given human nature	☐	☐	☐
Poor people get out of poverty through their own efforts	☐	☐	☐
I have experienced poverty	☐	☐	☐
Poverty is created, maintained and reproduced by social policies	☐	☐	☐
Many people make a living through poverty	☐	☐	☐
I would never let myself or my family become poor	☐	☐	☐
The welfare state has abolished poverty	☐	☐	☐
People drift into poverty through bad luck	☐	☐	☐
Poor people are more likely to be involved in criminal behaviour	☐	☐	☐
Poverty is a virtue	☐	☐	☐
Poverty is unacceptable	☐	☐	☐
Some poor people are blameless, others aren't	☐	☐	☐

Recommended reading

- Oppenheim C (1990) *Poverty: the facts*, London, Child Poverty Action Group.
A useful summary and analysis of poverty in modern Britain.

■ Blackburn C (1992) *Improving health and welfare work with families in poverty: A handbook*, Buckingham, Open University Press.

A useful and well designed team training handbook with exercises and information. The aim is to help health and welfare practitioners investigate the impact of poverty on the families they work with and to identify and plan strategies which address poverty. A structural explanation of poverty underpins the book. The intention is to enable practitioners to help families cope with and avoid the worst elements of poverty.

■ Blackburn C (1991) *Poverty and health: working with families*, Buckingham, Open University Press.

A companion volume to the above, which brings together recent research investigating the links between poverty and health.

■ Laughlin S and Black D (1995) *Poverty and health: Tools for change*, Birmingham, Public Health Alliance.

An excellent resource pack which comprehensively covers ideas, analysis, information and action. Included is a database which summarizes a variety of poverty and health projects.

■ Quick A and Wilkinson R (1991) *Income and health*, London, Socialist Health Association.

A short book which summarizes the evidence linking health and income and evidence which shows that inequalities damage health over and above the direct effects of poverty.

References

Amin K and Oppenheim C (1992) *Poverty in black and white: Deprivation and ethnic minorities*, London, Child Poverty Action Group.

Association of Community Health Councils for England and Wales (1990) *Health and wealth: A review of health inequalities in the UK*, London, Association of Community Health Councils for England and Wales.

Benzeval M, Judge K and Whitehead M (1995) *Tackling inequalities in health: An agenda for action*, London, The King's Fund.

Berthoud R, Lakey J and McKay S (1993) *The economic problems of disabled people*, London, Policy Studies Institute.

Blackburn C (1991) *Poverty and health: Working with families*, Buckingham, Open University Press.

Blackburn C (1992) *Improving health and welfare work with families in poverty: A handbook*, Buckingham, Open University Press.

Blackburn C (1993) "Making poverty a practice issue", *Health and Social Care*, **1,** 297–304.

Blane D, Brunner E and Wilkinson RG (1996) *Health and social organisation: Towards a health policy for the 21st century*, London, Routledge.

Boardman B (1991) *Fuel poverty*, London and New York, Bellhaven Press.

Bradshaw J and Holmes H (1989) *Living on the edge: A study of the living standards of families on benefit in Tyne and Wear*, Newcastle, Tyneside, Child Poverty Action Group. Tyneside.

Brown GW and Harris T (1978) *Social origins of depression*, London, Tavistock.

Cameron D and Jones IG (1985) An epidemiological and sociological analysis of the use of alcohol, tobacco and other drugs of solace, *Community Medicine*, **7,** 18–29.

Central Statistical Office (1994) *Social Trends 24*, London, HMSO.

Cohen S and Syme SL (eds) (1985) *Social support and health*, London, Academic Press.

Connelly J and Crown J (eds) (1994) *Homelessness and health*, London, Royal College of Physicians.

Crossan E and Amos A (1994) *Under a cloud*, Edinburgh, Health Education Board for Scotland.

Daykin N, Naidoo J and Wilson N (1995) *Effective health promotion in primary health care*, Bristol, Faculty of Health and Community Studies, University of the West of England.

Department of Health (1992) *The Health of the Nation: A strategy for health in England*, London, HMSO.

Department of Health (1993) *Better living, better lives*, London, HMSO.

Department of Health (1995) *Variations in health: What can the Department of Health and the NHS do? A report produced by the Variations sub-group of the Chief Medical Officer's Health of the Nation working group*, London, HMSO.

Department of Health (1997) *Target: Our Healthier Nation*, London, HMSO.

Department of Social Security (1992) *Households Below Average Income: A Statistical Analysis 1979–1988/9*, London, HMSO.

Dowler E and Calvert C (1995) *Nutrition and diet of lone-parent families in London*, London, Family Policy Study Centre.

Doyal L (1995) *What makes women sick? Gender and the political economy of health*, Basingstoke, Macmillan.

George V and Wilding P (1994) *Welfare and Ideology*, Hemel Hempstead, Harvester Wheatsheaf.

Glendinning C (1987) "Impoverishing women", in Walker A and Walker C (eds) *The Growing Divide: A Social Audit 1979–1987*, London, Child Poverty Action Group.

Glendinning C and Millar J (1992) *Women and poverty in Britain in the 1990s*, Brighton, Harvester Wheatsheaf.

Graham H (1987a) "Women's smoking and family health", *Social Science and Medicine*, **25**:1, 47–56.

Graham H (1987b) "Women's poverty and caring", in Glendinning C and Millar J (eds) *Women and poverty in Britain*, Brighton, Wheatsheaf.

Graham H (1993) *Hardship and health in women's lives*, Brighton, Harvester Wheatsheaf.

Graham H (1996) "Research on women and poverty: Trends and future directions", in Daykin

N and Lloyd L (eds) *Researching women, gender and health*, Bristol, Women and Health Research Group, University of the West of England.

Gregory J, Foster K, Tyler H and Wiseman M (1990) *The dietary and nutritional survey of British adults*, London, HMSO.

Harris CC (1991) "Recession, redundancy and age", in Brown P and Scase R (eds) *Poor Work: Disadvantage and the Division of Labour*, Buckingham, Open University Press.

HEA (1989) *Diet nutrition and healthy eating in low-income groups*, London, Health Education Authority.

HEA video (1991) "From boredom to boardroom: Helping ourselves to health; the Wirral women's experience", London, Health Education Authority.

House JS, Landis KR and Umberson D (1988) "Social relationships and health", *Science*, **241**, 540–45.

Laughlin S and Black D (1995) *Poverty and health: Tools for change*, Birmingham, Public Health Alliance.

Mack J and Lansley S (1985) *Poor Britain*, London, Allen and Unwin.

Madge N and Marmot MG (1987) Psychosocial factors in health, *Quarterly Journal of Social Affairs*, **3**(2): 81–134.

Marsh A and McKay S (1994) *Poor Smokers*, London, Policy Studies Institute.

NFA (1994) "Food and low income: A practical guide for advisers and supporters working with families and young people on low incomes", London, National Food Alliance.

Oppenheim C (1990) *Poverty: The Facts*, London, Child Poverty Action Group.

Richards D (1990) "Welfare rights advice as health provision", *Community Health Action*, **17** (Autumn Issue), 19–20.

Richards D (1993) *3 Year Report: Welfare Benefits Advice Service 1990–1993*.

Shiell A (1991) *Poverty and Inequalities in Health*, York, Centre for Health Economics.

Smaje C (1995) *"Health 'race' and ethnicity: Making sense of the evidence"*, London, Kings Fund Institute.

Standing Conference on Public Health Working Group Report (1994) *Housing, Homelessness and Health*, London, The Nuffield Provincial Hospitals Trust.

Townsend P (1979) *Poverty in the UK*, Harmondsworth, Penguin.

Townsend P, Davidson N and Whitehead M (1988) *Inequalities in Health: The Black Report and the Health Divide* (1987), Harmondsworth, Penguin.

Widgery D (1993) *Some lives! A GP's East End*, London, Simon and Schuster.

Wilkinson RG (1989) Class mortality differentials, income distribution and trends in poverty 1921–1981. *Journal of Social Policy*, **18:**3, 307–35.

Wilkinson RG (1993) "The impact of income inequality on life expectancy", in Platt S, Thomas H, Scott S and Williams G (eds) *Locating Health:*

Sociological and Historical Explorations, Aldershot, Avebury.

Wilkinson RG (1994) *"Unfair shares: The effects of widening income differences on the welfare of the young"*, London, Barnardos.

Wilkinson RG (1996) *Unhealthy societies: The afflictions of inequality*, London, Routledge.

Winyard S and Pond S (1989) *The case for a national minimum wage*, London, Low Pay Unit.

World Health Organization (1986) "Ottawa Charter for Health Promotion" *Journal of Health Promotion*, **1:** 1–4.

5 Targeting health promotion

Key points

- Targeting.
- The language of risk.
- Risk conditions.
- At-risk groups:
  - cultural essentialism and culture blaming;
  - universalism versus targeting.
- Risky behaviours:
  - assessment of risk;
  - the socio-cultural context of behaviour.
- Targeting as a professional and organizational strategy.

Overview

Targeting has become a key concept in health promotion. The term is used to describe several different activities. Targeting may be done in terms of diseases, lifecycles, lifestyles, social groups or social conditions. Targeting in terms of key diseases formed the basis of The "Health of the Nation" strategy (DoH, 1992). The revised strategy "Our Healthier Nation" goes beyond the disease-specific approach to look at population groups such as children, those of working age and the elderly as well as targeting inequalities (DoH, 1997). Targeting different stages of the lifecycle for preventive health action forms a central plank of primary health care provision (see Chapter 7 for further discussion of this kind of targeting).

Targeting lifestyles relies on a notion of health risk behaviours which are seen as the main targets for change by health promoters. This kind of targeting constructs certain behaviours as risky. Problems with this approach arise from the failure to place such behaviours in a social context. This chapter shows how epidemiological risk assessment is not shared by the general public, who adopt different means and measures of assessing risk. It has also been claimed that targeting lifestyles or behaviours may have the effect of maintaining or reinforcing inequalities in health. There are also ethical implications concerning the extension of health promotion into activities which are usually considered to be voluntary choices, e.g. diet, exercise patterns and the use of legal drugs such as alcohol and tobacco.

Targeting interventions towards specific groups such as ethnic minorities or young people is often advocated as a means of achieving equity. By directing activities towards groups most in need, health promoters seek to address inequalities in health. Targeting social conditions such as poverty (see Chapter 4) has been proposed as a preferred method of health promotion, but is an underdeveloped and underused strategy. This chapter examines the latter three forms of targeting and develops a critique against the wholesale adoption and application of a targeted approach in health promotion. We conclude by proposing a more considered approach to targeting which includes both its benefits and disadvantages.

What is targeting?

Health promotion is a huge area covering a multitude of activities. Targeting enables health promoters to focus on key areas instead of trying to do a little of everything. Targeting is central in health promotion policy, where it is valued as a means of establishing priorities and directing resources to effective interventions. Targeting is popular in part because it is seen as a means of implementing equity and channelling resources to those most at need. For health promoters who are concerned with equality and justice, targeting seems to offer the opportunity to develop practice which is in accordance with their values.

Targeting is carried out by many different agencies on the basis of a number of different criteria. Whilst targeting is often done on the basis of diseases or lifecycle stages, this chapter concentrates on targeting which is carried out according to three different criteria, namely lifestyles, social groups and social conditions.

The language of risk

The concept of targeting rests on a notion of risk. Epidemiologists assess risk in terms of the statistical probability of adverse events or death occurring. The link between this and certain identified factors can be expressed on a continuum from negligible to high. Lay people assess risk in the light of their personal experience and similarly may see actions as high or low risk, although this does not necessarily correspond with epidemiologists' assessment. Chapter 13 discusses the concept of risk in relation to accident prevention. The Chief Medical Officer has highlighted the importance of a common language of risk:

- **Hazard** – A set of circumstances which may have harmful consequences; a potential risk.
- **Risk assessment** – Usually expressed as the probability of an adverse event occurring in the population at risk.
- **Risk elimination** – May be the most effective course of action.

- **Risk management and control** – Generally done by a hazard analysis critical control point (HACCP) process which identifies critical points.
- **Risk–benefit analysis** – The weighing up of risks versus benefits of, e.g. medical treatment or leisure activities.

Table 5.1 *Risk of an individual dying or developing an adverse response in any one year*

Term used	Risk estimate	Example
High	Greater than 1:100	Mother–child transmission of HIV
Moderate	Between 1:100 and 1:1000	Smoking 10 cigarettes per day
Low	Between 1:1000 and 1:10,000	Road accident
Very low	Between 1:10,000 and 1:100,000	Leukaemia
Minimal	Between 1:100,000 and 1:1,000,000	Vaccination-associated polio
Negligible	Less than 1:1,000,000	Hit by lightning

Source: Calman (1996). Reproduced with permission

D The Chief Medical Officer has also identified the following terms which are important in any classification of risk:
- Avoidable–unavoidable
- Justifiable–unjustifiable
- Acceptable–unacceptable
- Serious–not serious

How would you define these terms and what examples would you give for each category?

Risk itself, defined as the likelihood of certain circumstances leading to undesirable health outcomes including disease and death, is used in several different ways.

Risk conditions, at-risk groups and risky behaviours

The above definitions refer primarily to the statistical likelihood of adverse reactions occurring. A different interpretation of risk and how it may be classified is given below in Figure 5.1.

Risk conditions

Risk may be used to refer to risk conditions, i.e. socially produced circumstances which, following the City of Toronto (1991), we term "risk conditions". The notion of risk conditions locates risk within social structures such as unemployment, pollution or income distribution. Poverty or homelessness thus viewed are social conditions which mean that certain people will inevitably experience these conditions. The individuals who are affected by these conditions may change, but if society is based around the maintenance and reproduction of these conditions, there will always be people who suffer from adverse social conditions.

Figure 5.1 *The relationship between risk and health (adapted from City of Toronto, 1991).*

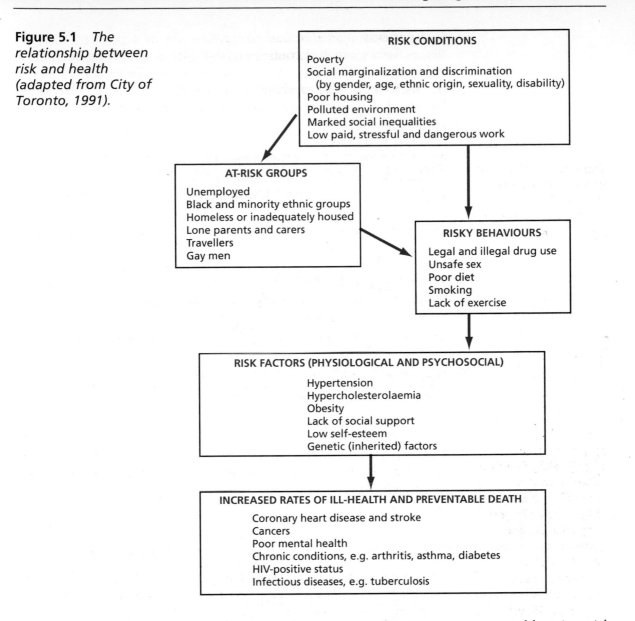

RISK CONDITIONS

Poverty
Social marginalization and discrimination
   (by gender, age, ethnic origin, sexuality, disability)
Poor housing
Polluted environment
Marked social inequalities
Low paid, stressful and dangerous work

AT-RISK GROUPS

Unemployed
Black and minority ethnic groups
Homeless or inadequately housed
Lone parents and carers
Travellers
Gay men

RISKY BEHAVIOURS

Legal and illegal drug use
Unsafe sex
Poor diet
Smoking
Lack of exercise

RISK FACTORS (PHYSIOLOGICAL AND PSYCHOSOCIAL)

Hypertension
Hypercholesterolaemia
Obesity
Lack of social support
Low self-esteem
Genetic (inherited) factors

INCREASED RATES OF ILL-HEALTH AND PREVENTABLE DEATH

Coronary heart disease and stroke
Cancers
Poor mental health
Chronic conditions, e.g. arthritis, asthma, diabetes
HIV-positive status
Infectious diseases, e.g. tuberculosis

As we saw in the previous chapter on poverty, addressing risk conditions demands broad-based policy changes. This approach has been endorsed by health promoters seeking to implement healthy public policy. Healthy public policy forms a central plank of health promotion theory (WHO, 1986), although rhetoric tends to outstrip action. Where attempts have been made, they tend to remain at the local level, e.g. in organizations, workplaces or local authorities. Chapter 8 discusses the concept of intersectoral collaboration and the difficulties in getting health to be seen as a political product and something that society, rather than individuals, can promote. A combination of material and ideological factors has led to the neglect of risk conditions in targeted health promotion activities.

Risk groups

Risk is used more commonly to refer to social groups deemed to be vulnerable to ill-health and premature death. Epidemiology identifies these groups on the basis of their physiological or behavioural factors, e.g. people with elevated serum cholesterol levels or people who smoke. Increasingly, health promotion has looked to research which identifies groups vulnerable to adverse health outcomes on the basis of psychosocial characteristics such as low income, homelessness or social isolation (Akehurst *et al.*, 1991; Hayes, 1992; McKie, 1994). The notion of risk groups, in contrast to the notion of risky behaviour, does recognize that such groups may not be able to change the circumstances which put them at risk. For example, people living in poor housing or on a low income are not generally perceived as able to voluntarily change these circumstances (see Chapter 4 for further discussion of promoting health in poverty).

Whilst there is a wealth of evidence to show that, in general, "at risk" groups correspond to people lacking in material and social resources, this approach suffers from the same problem of political unacceptability identified above. Whether the risk inheres in social conditions or in belonging to a group which is disadvantaged by these social conditions, the problem remains.

Risky behaviours

The most common use of risk in health promotion is in relation to certain activities deemed to be "risky behaviours" associated with negative health outcomes, for example excessive alcohol consumption, lack of physical exercise or smoking. This approach underpinned mainstream health promotion interventions, ranging from government policy initiatives such as "The Health of the Nation" (DoH, 1992), the approach taken in primary health care or national campaigns such as No Smoking Day.

> "The way in which people live and the lifestyles they adopt can have profound effects on subsequent health. Health education initiatives should continue to ensure that individuals are able to exercise informed choice when selecting the lifestyles which they adopt"
>
> (DoH, 1992:11).

Although the new Labour government has claimed that there has been an "excessive emphasis on lifestyle issues and the individual" (DoH, 1997:6), this approach is likely to continue. The notion of "risky behaviour" presupposes an element of volition. Health promotion activities directed at changing "risky behaviour" are based on the idea that people are able to change these behaviours, although there is debate about how this may be best achieved. The use of risky behaviours does not challenge the status quo; it locates the problem in certain people and it absolves the health promoter of the need to do more than point out the risks and advocate change.

The different kinds of targeting and uses of the term "risk" often overlap and are not always easy to disentangle. For example, smokers/smoking is often used interchangeably, although the former term targets a group whereas the latter term targets a behaviour. Social conditions and at risk groups may similarly be elided, e.g. poverty/poor people, whilst other terms include different categories of risk, e.g. illicit drug users.

Activity

List some categories of health risk. Do these categories refer to behaviour, groups, or social conditions? What are the implications and consequences of this for health promotion?

Conceptually however the different categories of targeting and risk are quite distinct, and we shall argue that the choice of targeting or risk category is significant and has important repercussions on the health promotion enterprise. We shall now examine these different types of targeting in greater detail.

Health promotion strategies

Targeting risky behaviour

Assessment of risk

Changing behaviour entails an assessment of risk. If individuals perceive a risk as serious and relevant, behaviour change is more likely (Becker, 1974). Yet people's assessment of risk is located within their own circumstances and priorities (Lupton, 1995; Graham, 1996). Personal circumstances may mean that individuals weight epidemiological risks differently, for example, the risks associated with drug taking may be justified by the more urgent need to cope with daily stresses.

R Do you engage in any behaviours which you know are bad for your health? What is your reason for continuing with these behaviours?

Davison *et al.* (1992) explore the basis for the difference between epidemiological and individual risk assessment using the example of coronary heart disease. They argue that epidemiology correlates "misfortune" or the occurrence of disease with risk behaviours. Individuals explain "misfortune" with reference to the circumstances of people they know or have heard about. Epidemiological assessment gives rise to the notion of "candidates" or people who exhibit risk behaviours. Individuals talk of "victims" of early death or disease. It might be expected that these two assessments of risk would coincide.

R   Can you think of examples where a "candidate" for ill-health lived to a ripe old age? Or where a "victim" was a paragon of healthy lifestyles?
What is the effect of such anomalies?

Lay perceptions of risk are affected by many factors other than epidemiological risk assessment. Social or cultural norms may suggest that some behaviours which carry risks are expected and valued. For example, heavy drinking amongst young men and smoking amongst young people are behaviours which are known to be influenced by peer pressure (Brynin and Scott, 1996). Risks associated with illegal or deviant behaviour are perceived as greater than risks associated with legal or acceptable behaviour. For example, deaths due to ecstasy taking at raves are far less than deaths and accidents due to youthful alcohol consumption, yet it is the former which attracts most attention and coverage.

People's assessment of the value of behavioural changes takes place within a social and cultural context in which they balance their long-term risk against immediate functions and gratification. Behavioural change is difficult to achieve and health promoters' assurances of health benefits may not be immediately apparent. The immediate benefits of behaviours known to carry health risks (e.g. smoking or high fat, high sugar diets) may outweigh the long-term risks (Charles and Kerr, 1986; Graham, 1987).

D   What are the implications for health promotion of taking into account lay perceptions of risk?

The complexity of risk assessment and attribution suggests that, in order to be effective, health promotion needs to have a wide range of strategies at its disposal. In practice, health promotion strategies prove to be rather narrow in scope and beset by problems. Addressing risk behaviours tends to result in simple behavioural messsages such as "eat less salt" or "eat less saturated fat". However the wider social and cultural context in which behaviours are formed, maintained and reproduced is ignored. In the case of diet this includes commercial pressures to consume convenience food high in fat and salt and government policies on food production.

The problems of addressing behaviour in a vacuum have not led to health promotion abandoning the behaviour change approach. Instead, behaviour change is increasingly recognized as difficult to achieve, leading to a corresponding lowering of expectations. Prochaska and DiClemente's (1984) cycle of change model, which enables health promoters to locate people in terms of their readiness to change, has been widely adopted. Part of its popularity is that it encourages a tailored intervention for each individual. It is also popular, however, because it suggests that if people are not ready for change, health promoters need do no more than perhaps repeat the assessment in the future. The model says nothing about why some people find it harder than others to change, or the role the environment plays in behavioural choices.

It has been argued that targeting risky behaviours may lead to a widening of present health inequalities (Raymond, 1989; McKie, 1994). This is because people who have sufficient material and emotional resources find behavioural change much easier than people coping with straitened circumstances. The national reduction in smoking rates has been achieved by the higher social classes, whilst smoking rates of the most impoverished groups has shown no equivalent reduction (Marsh and McKay, 1994). Claims that behavioural change targets have been achieved may mask the fact that this is because the health of the most advantaged groups has improved, leaving disadvantaged groups trailing further behind than before (Wilkinson, 1994).

D Increasing taxes on tobacco has been shown to reduce smoking rates but it is also criticized as representing a further financial burden for the poor who cannot break the habit (Marsh and Mackay, 1994). Can you think of other examples where addressing risk behaviours merely widens inequalities in health?

It is apparent and noteworthy that by using epidemiological data certain types of behaviour are targeted and other types of behaviour, equally relevant to health, are not. Chapter 2 explores further this issue of how risk is framed within research. Private car use is a good example of a health-related behaviour which has largely escaped the attention of health promoters. Figure 5.2 shows how private car use could be constructed as a targeted risk behaviour. The huge commercial and economic interests invested in the car industry provide one obvious reason for its relative invisibility as a health issue. Added to this is the political influence of the road lobby and the huge amount of government revenue derived from petrol and car tax. A further factor is the social approval afforded to private car use, and the fact that "those people with the power to do so are themselves likely to have a 'lifestyle' in which the motor car plays a prominent role" (Hunt, 1993:248). The relationship between transport policies and health is discussed in Chapter 10 on coronary heart disease and stroke.

Targeting risk groups

If targeting risky behaviours is fraught with problems, does targeting at-risk groups fare any better? At first sight it seems an attractive proposition. Resources may be directed towards groups with the highest levels of health needs, which should prove both effective and equitable. Targeting at-risk groups may therefore appeal to health promoters who are concerned with issues of equity.

Risk groups may be defined on the basis of psychosocial, cultural or biological risk factors. Psychosocial risk factors include unemployment, low self-esteem and low levels of social support. Groups may be identified as "at-risk" because their circumstances mean they find it difficult to access services, e.g. homeless people. Cultural norms may be used to target particular groups, e.g. ethnic minority groups' cultures (rather than their socially disadvantaged status) have been the target of health education campaigns on diet and exercise. Such targeting is based on a notion of "cultural essentialism" which reduces complex behaviour and socio-economic environments to cultural norms.

Biological risk factors include genetically acquired factors and physical health status, e.g. people with inherited blood disorders,

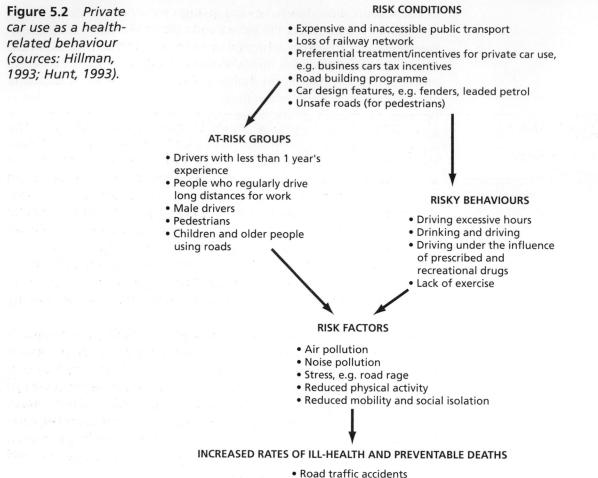

Figure 5.2 *Private car use as a health-related behaviour (sources: Hillman, 1993; Hunt, 1993).*

RISK CONDITIONS

• Expensive and inaccessible public transport
• Loss of railway network
• Preferential treatment/incentives for private car use, e.g. business cars tax incentives
• Road building programme
• Car design features, e.g. fenders, leaded petrol
• Unsafe roads (for pedestrians)

AT-RISK GROUPS

• Drivers with less than 1 year's experience
• People who regularly drive long distances for work
• Male drivers
• Pedestrians
• Children and older people using roads

RISKY BEHAVIOURS

• Driving excessive hours
• Drinking and driving
• Driving under the influence of prescribed and recreational drugs
• Lack of exercise

RISK FACTORS

• Air pollution
• Noise pollution
• Stress, e.g. road rage
• Reduced physical activity
• Reduced mobility and social isolation

INCREASED RATES OF ILL-HEALTH AND PREVENTABLE DEATHS

• Road traffic accidents
• Asthma

asthmatics and diabetics. At-risk groups are usually defined in relation to a specific health issue, e.g. gay men and HIV, travelling families and accidents, homeless people and tuberculosis.

D What problems might there be in defining risk groups in these ways?

Groups are assumed to be homogenous when they may be mixed in terms of other important characteristics such as social class or gender. Groups defined as at risk of certain conditions tend to have their broader and more significant health problems minimized and neglected. For example, African–Caribbeans may be recognized as at risk of sickle cell disease, but their higher risk of stroke, hypertension, diabetes, mental ill-health and accidents (Ahmad, 1993) tends to be invisible. Finally, constructing at-risk groups in this way also runs the risk of "culture blaming", that is, the group's cultural norms may be blamed for their increased risk, and viewed as deviant or deficient. The following case studies illustrate some of the dilemmas in targeting risk groups. In the first, the Asian rickets campaign of the early 1980s shows how targeting can result in groups being blamed for their condition. The second case study shows how targeting people with sickle cell and thalassaemia can ensure that a condition is fully addressed. The third case study focuses on whether attempts to reduce the spread of HIV should be targeted at gay men.

Case study

Asian rickets campaign

This campaign has been extensively documented (Sheiham and Quick, 1982; Douglas, 1995; Pearson, 1986) and provides an interesting example of the pitfalls which may arise when at-risk groups are targeted. The campaign was launched by the Department of Health as a result of medical observations that rickets, a vitamin D deficiency disease, was reappearing amongst Asian children. A health education campaign which focused on messages advocating dietary change and increased exposure of the skin to sunlight was launched. Asian parents were advised to eat foods rich in vitamin D such as oily fish and margarine and to let their children play in the sun. Leaflets and posters were translated into the main Asian community languages.

Asian community leaders responded angrily, saying the campaign was an attack on cultural norms and used a notion of cultural essentialism, whereby the risk behaviour (low vitamin D intake) was constructed as an attribute of Asian culture and diet. A better course of action, it was suggested, would have been to fortify a dietary staple food, such as chapatti flour. This had been the government response to rickets the first time round, in the 1950s, when vitamin D had been added to margarine, dried milk and cereals. Dietary fortification had proved to be a successful strategy.

This case study demonstrates the need for cultural sensitivity and partnership if at-risk groups are to be targeted. The Asian rickets campaign was a top-down intervention. Its messages were interpreted as victim blaming, as placing the blame for rickets within a deficient culture. The campaign advocated playing in the open air and changing diets without recognizing the important reasons why these behaviours may not be adopted (e.g. fears for safety in public areas or the cultural significance of diet). The Asian rickets campaign also provides an example of inconsistency in government policy. When rickets was perceived as a general health problem affecting the public, dietary fortification was implemented. When rickets became an Asian problem, affecting minority ethnic groups, health education was advocated as a sufficient government response. The campaign was seen therefore as an example of ethnocentricity and dual standards (Sheiham and Quick, 1982; Pearson, 1986; Douglas, 1995).

Case study *Sickle cell and thalassaemia*	The example of sickle cell and thalassaemia illustrates how targeting may be used to achieve inclusion and the provision of appropriate services within the healthcare sector.

> "Sickle cell anaemia is not of great consequence to us in the context of genetic counselling in the United Kingdom. The sickling trait and sickle cell anaemia appear to be confined to peoples of African and Eastern origin."
>
> (Stevenson and Davison, cited in Anionwu, 1993.)

Sickle cell disorders and thalassaemia are inherited blood disorders which mainly affect Black and minority ethnic groups, and are therefore excluded from the wider health agenda. Asian cultures, in this instance the practice of consanguinous marriages, have been blamed for causing the problem. Sickle cell and thalassaemia are associated with painful crises and life-threatening infections. A conservative estimate of the number of affected people in Britain is 5000 – similar to the number of people affected by the inherited conditions of haemophilia and cystic fibrosis. Testing for the condition is cheap and simple. Voluntary national support organizations were founded in the 1970s, OSCAR (Organization for Sickle Cell Action and Research) in 1975, the UK Thalassaemia Society in 1976 and the Sickle Cell Society in 1979. These organizations provide a variety of services including advice, education and counselling as well as lobbying for national mainstream provision of services within the NHS. Provision of sickle cell and thalassaemia services remains patchy throughout the country. There is no national screening programme for these blood disorders, although such a programme is provided for phenylketonuria, which affects 10–12 babies per 100,000. For comparison, 500 plus per 100,000 babies of African–Caribbean origin are affected by sickle cell disease (Anionwu, 1993).

This example of sickle cell disorders and thalassaemia shows how significant, predictable and treatable risk may remain largely invisible as long as it is perceived as being relevant only to minority groups. Targeting those at risk from these conditions is a means of achieving inclusion into mainstream health agendas.

The following case study of gay men and HIV/AIDS health education illustrates the tensions and dilemmas of targeting risk groups versus universalism or the whole population approach.

Case study *Gay men and HIV/AIDS*	**Stages in the response to HIV: from targeting to universalism and back** **1981–82** In the USA, the first deaths from AIDS are recognized following reports of gay men dying from pneumonia and Kaposi's sarcoma.

Hypotheses that the disease was related to gay lifestyles led to AIDS being referred to as GRID – gay related immune deficiency. The '4Hs' hypothesis identified four at-risk groups – homosexuals, heroin addicts, Haitians and haemophiliacs.

1983
- HIV isolated.
- In the USA, gay men publish a 40-page booklet of safer sex guidelines.
- In the UK, the Medical Research Council sets up a working party on AIDS. The Terrence Higgins Trust (THT) is set up as a self-help group.

1984
In the UK the Public Health and Control of Diseases Act establishes a blood screening programme (at a cost of £4 million) and enables powers to detain and hospitalize PWAs (people with AIDS). The THT telephone help line is set up.

1985
The government allocates £135,000 for education and prevention.
The THT receives some government funding and the UK government sets up an Expert Advisory Group on AIDS. There is a communion wine scare in the media after a prison chaplain dies from AIDS. HIV antibody testing becomes widely available in the UK.

1986
A report by the USA's Surgeon-General identifies a potential heterosexually transmitted epidemic, leading to a new sense of urgency in official circles.
The UK government's HIV/AIDS budget is set at £20 million. The government launches its "Don't aid AIDS campaign".

1987
The national "Don't die of ignorance" HIV/AIDS campaign is launched in the UK. The government sets up an all party Social Services Committee to investigate. The government gives the THT £466,000 and a £10 million *ex gratia* payment to the Haemophilia Society to set up a trust fund for HIV-positive haemophiliacs.
The activist group ACTUP (AIDS Coalition To Unleash Power) is set up in New York, USA.
The first conference on women and AIDS is held in London.

1988
Section 28 of the UK Local Government Act, which directs local authorities not to promote homosexuality as a "pretended family relationship" has the effect of scaring teachers off sex education which acknowledges homosexuality.

1989

The Health Education Authority (HEA) places safer sex adverts in the gay and lesbian press for the first time, at a cost of 3% of the £10 million AIDS education budget. The HEA launches its first major advertising campaign targeted at women.

The government stops funding the THT's health education activities.

1990

The HEA launches its MESMAC (men who have sex with men: action in the community) project.

Re-gaying AIDS conference is held in Amsterdam.

UK statistics show that heterosexuals infected by HIV rose by 61% during the year, compared to an increase of 42% among gay or bisexual men. However those affected are still predominantly gay or bisexual (3295 gay or bisexual men, 1237 heterosexual men and women).

1992

A UK report finds that of 226 agencies with a remit for HIV prevention (mostly in the statutory sector), only one third had ever targeted gay men.

The Advisory Group to the HEA's MESMAC project resign *en masse*, protesting that their advice has been ignored.

1993

Following reports that Brighton has the highest rate of HIV infection and AIDS deaths, FAB is established as a self-help group with some health authority funding. FAB's health promotion material is seized by police, and the health authority withdraws funding.

1994

Epidemiological assessment shows that sex between men is the largest risk category amongst reported HIV infection cases, accounting for 60% of the cumulative total and 57% of the 2597 reports received in the twelve months up to April 1994.

1996

Ring fenced money for HIV/AIDS ends. Funding for HIV/AIDS organizations in the voluntary sector is under threat.

(Sources: Wilton, 1992; King, 1993; Public Health Laboratory Service Communicable Diseases Surveillance Centre, 1994; Patton, 1994; Richardson, 1994; BBC, 1995.)

Gay men and intravenous drug users were the inital target of HIV/AIDS health education messages in the early 1980s. Alongside the success of this approach in reducing the HIV infection rate amongst gay men were negative effects such as the maintenance of heterosexuals' illusion of invulnerability and a homophobic backlash.

Predictions in the mid-1980s of a heterosexual epidemic led to a change in emphasis. By 1990 the health education message had changed to "it's not who you are but what you do", i.e. targeting risky behaviour rather than risk groups. This was accompanied by a shift in funding from gay projects towards professionally-led initiatives aimed at the heterosexual population.

> "The government response to AIDS was largely shaped by the political necessity of being seen to do something for the general public (read, 'heterosexuals') while continuing to insist on the deviant status of homosexuality, extramarital sex and injecting drug use . . ."
>
> (Wilton, 1992:110).

The MESMAC (men who have sex with men: action in the community) project recognized the fluidity of sexual identity and sought to reach men who did not necessarily identify as gay but had sex with men, for example in public sex environments. The professional and official takeover of HIV/AIDS health promotion work led to significant changes in strategies and messages. Targeting was replaced by a whole population or universalist approach, exemplified by the mass media campaigns and household leaflet drop of 1987. Everyone was deemed to be at risk.

D List the advantages and disadvantages of a universalist approach to HIV/AIDS.

Grass roots activism among the gay community was replaced by big budget mass media advertising. The explicit advice contained in safer sex literature for gay men was deemed to be unsuitable and offensive for the general public. New messages, informed by a New Right moral agenda, focused on monogamy and a range of advice on risk reduction.

Small scale community initiatives had been successful in instigating safer sex practices among gay men, but gay men's groups went along with this shift to mainstreaming HIV work because it was tied in to mainstream funding and was seen as a means of avoiding stigmatization and marginalization. The whole tone of HIV education changed. Whereas gay activists advocated minimal behavioural change and were concerned to provide sex-positive messages, these principles were abandoned once professional health promoters entered the arena.

> "... gay health educators have felt both an ethical and a practical imperative to cause only the minimum necessary disruption to gay men's sexual practices in the interests of reducing or preventing HIV transmission"
>
> (King, 1993:149).

With hindsight, it has been argued that the "de-gaying" of HIV/AIDS has had profoundly negative effects on the group which remains at highest risk of infection.

This has led to more recent calls to "re-gay AIDS" and to re-allocate resources to the gay community which is still bearing the major burden of HIV infection and its consequences. Another factor is the fear that young gay men new to the scene are missing out on safer sex messages. There has also been a breakdown of grassroots gay organizations and networks, caused by the professionalization of HIV health education and the "burning out" of many activists. Targeting may be seen as a means of increasing professional power.

Activity

Consider the following arguments for and against targeting in the case of gay men and HIV.
Which view is closest to your own?
Try to argue for one of these positions with a colleague.

- HIV affects everyone. It's vital that all sexually active people recognize the importance of practising safer sex. It is particular behaviours, not belonging to a particular group, which transmits HIV. The best means to protect the rights of HIV-positive people is by ensuring that everyone realizes they are potentially at risk.

- In Britain, HIV predominantly affects gay men. Messages and resources need to be directed towards gay men and men who have sex with men. In the 1980s gay men adopted safer sex on a wide scale, demonstrating how effective health education can be. Awareness of safer sex within the gay community needs reinforcement, especially for younger gay men and men new to being gay.

A targeted approach means that efforts may be directed towards gay men who are still at disproportionate risk of HIV infection. Some sections of the gay community may be relatively easily reached through their involvement in "the scene". But other gay men, unless they are specifically targeted, are unlikely to be reached; in particular, young gay men and men who have sex in public sex environments. Chapter 13 discusses a resource for gay men in relationships but who may have sex with other partners. During the 1980s there were significant changes in sexual behaviour among gay men (King, 1993), demonstrating that targeted campaigns are effective. Re-establishing and consolidating safer sex as a social and cultural norm is more feasible within the gay community than within heterosexual society. The broader health promotion policy framework (DoH, 1992) identifies HIV/AIDS but does not specifically target gay men or HIV-positive people.

Several different tensions surround the issue of targeting at-risk groups. Ideally, targeting should supplement a universal infrastructure, guaranteeing sensitive information and services. In the real world, the needs of specific at-risk groups are often ignored in universal health service provision, with the result that targeting appears to be the only means of guaranteeing that minimum health needs are met. This is the argument advanced in the case of sickle cell and thalassaemia.

On the other hand, specific health needs of identified minority groups are at risk of being marginalized and stigmatized unless there is a universal health promotion programme. This is demonstrated by the Asian rickets campaign and the case study of gay men and HIV/AIDS. Gay men's organizations accepted a universal strategy because they thought that if HIV/AIDS was perceived as a general health problem, applicable to everyone, homophobic attitudes and policies would have the ground cut from under them. The strength of universalism is inclusion. Yet the history of gay men and HIV/AIDS shows that, paradoxically, universalism can go hand-in-hand with exclusionary policies and ideology. By constructing HIV/AIDS as a general (heterosexual) health problem, the fact that gay men were, and continue to be, disproportionately at risk, was ignored. Universalism led to a reallocation of resources, away from the groups most at need.

In practice then, the sound reasons for targeting at-risk groups – a concern with equity and effectiveness – are not always achieved. Targeting at-risk groups is no guarantee that health inequalities will be addressed or reduced, or that health promotion interventions will prove more effective than a whole population approach.

Targeting risk conditions

In the light of the many problems and dilemmas associated with targeting risky behaviours or at-risk groups outlined above, would targeting risk conditions be a better strategy to pursue? Targeting risk conditions appears to provide a solution to some dilemmas, e.g. the dangers of individual or culture blaming, and focusing on symptoms instead of causes of ill-health. Social-structural, economic and physical conditions are independent of the people who experience them and are known to be closely correlated with health outcomes. There is a significant body of health promotion theory which utilizes this analysis, most notably the WHO's Health for All 2000 programme and Charter for Health Promotion (WHO, 1979, 1986), and a number of interventions which seek to put this into practice, e.g. the Sheffield Health programme (Halliday, 1991).

D What risk conditions would you identify as areas to target?

It is interesting to note that whereas risky behaviours and at-risk groups are common terms in health promotion, risk conditions is not. Health promotion is driven by epidemiological risk factors which highlight medical conditions and diseases. As we saw in Chapter 2, a social epidemiology which highlights the links between social structures, policy and health is only now emerging. In Chapter 4 we saw how targeting poverty is an overtly political activity which challenges existing policy and may seem beyond the remit of health promoters.

Conclusion

Targeting health promotion is based on notions of risk which prove problematic in practice. Health promotion most commonly defines risk as a property of behaviour or lifestyles. There are several reasons why the notion of risky behaviours is popular. It is scientifically based, with a body of epidemiological evidence to support its causal role in the aetiology of disease and the efficacy of change in reducing risk. It provides a peg upon which individual advice and information can be given, fitting it to the client basis of much health promotion work. Behavioural change is the voluntary exercise of individual choice and does not impinge on individual freedom or responsibility.

There are, however, problems with such an approach. The lack of congruence between epidemiologically defined risk behaviours and the lay perception of such behaviour creates immediate problems of relevance and acceptance. Behaviour itself is viewed as being either individually and voluntarily chosen, or inherent in certain cultural or social groups' norms. This all too easily leads to individual or culture blaming. The broader economic and social context which influences health-related behaviours is down-played. A focus on behaviour change does not impact on health inequalities, since it is the most advantaged people who find it easiest to change their behaviour.

Targeting at-risk groups, which at first sight might appear both more equitable and more effective, is also problematic. Targeting at-risk groups can easily become an exercise in culture-blaming. Targeting is often used as a substitute for universalism and may become a means of avoiding, instead of supplementing, mainstream provision. Targeting has become part of the professional repertoire of health promoters, and may serve to reinforce professional power at the expense of empowering individuals or communities.

Targeting risk conditions appears to offer a way out of these dilemmas. Focusing on the underlying social, political, economic and environmental conditions which pose risks for specific groups offers the chance to "travel upstream" and address risk as a manageable property of institutions and policies. This provides a means of separating risk from individual- or culture-blaming and social stereotyping.

There are good reasons for the popularity of targeting. However, analysis of examples of targeted health promotion activities demonstrates that these laudable aims are often not achieved in practice. In addition, it has been pointed out that many major improvements in public health have been achieved without targeting (Ingledew, 1989;

McKie, 1994). The wholesale application of targeting may not represent the best means of promoting health. By considering in a more critical manner the benefits and problems of targeting, and through the analytical separation of the different categories of risk subsumed under the notion of targeting, health promoters may arrive at a more balanced evaluation of the practice of targeting. The intention of this chapter is to enable health promoters to undertake this analysis and acquire a more critical understanding of the dilemmas and tensions which exist in targeted activities.

Further discussion

- How can health promoters ensure that they incorporate the principle of equity in their practice? Is targeting an effective way to achieve this?
- How might health promotion interventions targeted at specific at-risk groups avoid falling into the traps of cultural essentialism and stereotyping?
- Who stands to gain most from targeting – organizations, health promoters, or clients?

D

The Labour government has stated that whilst targeting in terms of risk factors and diseases is useful, it also intends to target population groups such as children and older people. What are the advantages and disadvantages of targeting population groups rather than risk factors and diseases?

Recommended reading

- McKie L (1994) *Risky behaviours – healthy lifestyles*, Lancaster, Quay Publishing Limited.
  A readable and comprehensive account of the debate surrounding the notion of risk and how this feeds into health promotion.

- Evans B, Sansberg S and Watson S (eds) (1992) *Working where the risks are: Issues in HIV prevention*, London, Health Education Authority.
  A discussion of HIV prevention among risk groups including gay men, drug users, young people and Black and minority ethnic communities.

- Douglas J (1995) "Developing anti-racist health promotion strategies", in Burrows R, Nettleton S and Burrows R (eds), *The sociology of health promotion*, pp. 70–77, London, Routledge.
  A critique of health promotion's targeting of Black and minority ethnic groups.

■ Calman K (1996) "On the state of the public health", *Health Trends*, **28**:3, 79–88.
Includes a discussion on the language of risk with suggestions for terminology.

References

Ahmad WI (1993) *"Race" and health in contemporary Britain*, Buckingham, Open University Press.

Anionwu EN (1993) "Sickle cell and thalassaemia: community experiences and official response", in Ahmad WIU (ed.) *"Race" and health in contemporary Britain*, Buckingham, Open University Press.

Akehurst R, Godfrey C, Hutton J and Robertson E (1991) *"The Health of the Nation", An economic perspective on target setting Discussion Paper 92*, York, Centre for Health Economics, University of York.

Becker MH (ed.) (1974) *The health belief model and personal health behaviour*, Thorofare, New Jersey, Slack.

BBC (1995) *Fine cut: The end of innocence*, BBC2 5/12/95.

Brynin M and Scott J (1996) *Young people, health and the family*, London, Health Education Authority.

Calman K (1996) "On the state of the public health", *Health Trends*, **28**(3), 79–88.

Charles N and Kerr M (1986) "Issues of responsibility and control in the feeding of families", in Rodmell S and Watt A (eds) *The politics of health education: Raising the issues*, London, Routledge and Kegan Paul.

City of Toronto Community Health Information Section (1991) *Health inequalities in the city of Toronto: Summary Report*, Toronto, Department of Public Health.

Davison C, Frankel S and Davey Smith G (1992) "The limits of lifestyle: Re-assessing 'fatalism' in the popular culture of illness prevention", *Social Science and Medicine*, **34**(6), 675–85.

Department of Health (1992) *The Health of the Nation: A strategy for health in England*, London, HMSO.

Department of Health (1997) *Target: Our Healthier Nation*, London, HMSO.

Douglas J (1995) "Developing anti-racist health promotion strategies", in Burrows R, Nettleton S and Burrows R (eds) *The sociology of health promotion*, pp. 70–77, London, Routledge.

Graham H (1987) "Women's smoking and family health", *Social Science and Medicine*, **25**, 47–56.

Graham H (1996) "Research on women and poverty: Trends and future directions", in Daykin N and Lloyd L (eds) *Researching women, gender and health*, Bristol, Women and Health Research Group, University of the West of England.

Halliday M (1991) *Our city, our health*, Sheffield, Healthy Sheffield.

Hayes MV (1992) "On the epistemology of risk: Language, logic and social science", *Social Science and Medicine*, **35**(4), 401–7.

Hillman M (1993) "Social goals for transport policy", in Beattie A *et al.* (eds) *Health and wellbeing: A reader*, pp. 237–47, Basingstoke, Macmillan.

Hunt SM (1993) "The public health implications of private cars", in Beattie A *et al.* (eds) *Health and wellbeing: A reader*, pp. 248–56, Basingstoke, Macmillan.

Ingledew D (1989) "Target setting for the health of populations: Some observations", *Health Promotion*, **4**(4), 357–69.

Lupton D (1995) *The imperative of health: Public health and the regulated body*, London, Sage.

King E (1993) *Safety in numbers: Safer sex and gay men*, London, Cassell.

Marsh A and McKay S (1994) *Poor smokers*, London, Policy Studies Institute.

McKie L (1994) *Risky behaviours – healthy lifestyles*, Lancaster, Quay Publishing Limited.

Patton C (1994) *Last served? Gendering the HIV pandemic*, London, Taylor and Francis.

Pearson M (1986) "Racist notions of ethnicity and culture in health education", in Rodmell S and Watt A (eds) *The politics of health education*, London, Routledge and Kegan Paul.

Plant M and Plant M (1992) *Risk-takers: alcohol, drugs, sex and youth*, London and New York, Tavistock/Routledge.

Prochaska JO and DiClemente C (1984) *The trans-theoretical approach: Crossing traditional foundations of change*, Homewood, Ill., Don Jones/Irwin.

Public Health Laboratory Service Communicable Disease Surveillance Centre (1994) *Communicable disease report*, London, PHLS.

Raymond JS (1989) "Behavioral epidemiology: The science of health promotion", *Health Promotion*, 4(4), 281–86.

Richardson D (1994) "AIDS: Issues for feminism in the UK", in Doyal L, Naidoo J and Wilton T (eds) *AIDS: Setting a feminist agenda*, pp. 42–57, London, Taylor and Francis.

Sheiham H and Quick A (1982) *The rickets report*, London, Haringey CHC and CRC.

Wilkinson RG (1994) *Unfair shares: The effects of widening income differences on the welfare of the young*, London, Barnardos.

Wilton T (1992) *Antibody politic: AIDS and society*, Cheltenham, New Clarion Press.

WHO (1978) *Report on the primary health care conference: Alma Ata*, Geneva, WHO.

WHO (1985) *Targets for health for all*, Copenhagen, WHO, Regional Office for Europe.

WHO (1986) "Ottawa Charter for health promotion", *Journal of Health Promotion*, **1**, 1–4.

6 Marketing health

Overview

We live in a society in which a vast array of products is successfully marketed using sophisticated methods. People are persuaded to buy items they never thought they would need. Social marketing is concerned with the introduction and dissemination of ideas and issues. Its techniques are being widely adopted in health promotion in order to maximize access to target groups and influence the acceptability of healthy lifestyles. This chapter discusses the argument that there are basic similarities between marketing and health promotion. Marketing is a sophisticated method of targeting which involves the consumer or client and gives them some control over the development of health messages, whilst health promotion also seeks to involve and empower people.

The recognition that the commercial world has been remarkably successful in its use of marketing has prompted health promoters to question whether there are lessons to be learnt. If marketing can sell products and lifestyles which create ill-health, such as confectionery, tobacco and fast cars or use "health" to sell a wide variety of apparently unrelated products from sanitary towels to breakfast cereals, perhaps health promoters can use marketing techniques to package health in a way which makes it more desirable. This chapter discusses the ethical implications of "selling health" and debates whether marketing principles and health promotion are compatible.

Introduction

The provision of information about healthy lifestyles and services has long been considered a crucial part of health promotion. Reaching people through the mass media has therefore been a major activity. The belief that the mass media could provide a panacea for health promoters in which they could convey a health message to huge numbers of people who would then be persuaded to change their behaviour has been tempered by numerous research studies (Tones and Tilford, 1994, provides a useful summary). Most of these studies suggest that the mass media can be successful in raising awareness of health issues and enhancing motivation to change amongst those already positively disposed to do so:

> "It is relatively easy to agenda set and communicate simple information; it is increasingly difficult to change attitudes, teach complex skills and persuade people to adopt new behaviours especially where these involve exertion, discomfort or the abandoning of pleasure"
>
> (Tones and Tilford, 1994:182).

Interpersonal support and advice is, however, necessary to help people to make decisions about any change in their behaviour. People need to be actively involved – articulating their concerns, setting goals, discussing how changes can be made – and this can only be done in two-way communication which is tailored to the needs of a specific individual or group. The recognition that mass media advertising has little direct effect on people's behaviour has led health promoters to look to the world of commerce to find out how marketing identifies and reaches targeted audiences for specific products.

Social marketing

R What do you understand by the term marketing?

For most people, marketing is synonymous with advertising and selling and implies being persuaded to buy something which they may not necessarily want or need. For many health practitioners, health promotion is seen in the same way as involving promotional tactics of "pushing" or "selling" a health message to people who may be resistant (Williams, 1985; Downie *et al.*, 1990). Underpinning this is the assumption that just as people choose products, people choose health behaviours and that their choices can be influenced.

The term social marketing was first used in 1971 by Kotler and Zaltman who described it as:

> "the design, implementation and control of programs calculated to influence the acceptability of social ideas and involving considerations of product, planning, pricing, communication, distribution and marketing research."

They argued that just as there is a marketplace for products, there is a marketplace for ideas and the same techniques which are used to sell products can be used to sell an idea or cause or to persuade, influence or motivate people to change their behaviour or use a service. The process is based on the concept of a mutually beneficial exchange. In commercial terms, the consumer gets a product they want at a price they can afford and the producer gets a profit. In the

D What benefit does the health promoter get from the exchange?

marketing of health, the consumer gets the promise of improved health and quality of life at a possible cost of giving up a pleasure (e.g. chocolate, cigarettes) or making some physical or psychological effort (e.g. going to a gym).

According to Hastings and Haywood (1991) commercial marketing is "essentially about getting the right product, at the right price, in the right place at the right time presented in such a way as to successfully satisfy the needs of the consumer". The whole process thus needs to be carefully researched and planned. The needs and values of the market or the audience have to be analysed, a message developed which will appeal to the particular market segment which is being targeted and the message tested among representatives of the target group. Opinions of influential leaders may be sought before the message is promoted using channels of communication appropriate to the target group. Flora and Lefebvre (1988) propose the following components of social marketing (Table 6.1).

Table 6.1 *The components of social marketing*

- Consumer orientation
- Identification of key target audience through segmentation and analysis
- Voluntary and mutually beneficial exchange
- Formative research
- Clear objective setting
- Channel analysis
- A marketing mix of product, price, place and promotion
- Monitoring and evaluation

D How might the techniques and principles in Table 6.1 be useful in health promotion?

The market

A central tenet of marketing is a consumer orientation: an understanding of the perceptions, motivations, behaviour and needs of people which enables the message to be matched to the audience (Hastings and Haywood, 1991). A message such as "Quitting is Winning" is directed towards all smokers, but the population of smokers is made up of numerous subgroups which differ in a variety of ways. We saw in Chapter 5 that where messages are tailored or targeted it is usually on the basis of professional perceptions of risk and thus relates to epidemiological and demographic classifications. People are also differentiated by their consumption patterns (just as they are by social variables). Marketing is based on the recognition and identification of different groups of people or "market segments". These groups are like each other and differ from other groups according to a whole range of finely detailed psychographic and lifestyle attributes and characteristics such as degree of conformity, ambition or risk taking.

D In Table 6.2 can you identify which are the male profiles and which the female? Can you see any difficulties with targeting health promotion to such defined groups?

Table 6.2 *Psychographic profiles: A large scale study of the personalities, aspirations and social roles of American men and women identified the following distinct psychographic profiles*

The quiet family person	The conformist
The traditionalist	The drudge
The discontent	The natural contented
The ethical highbrow	The indulger
The pleasure oriented	The free spender
The achiever	The puritan
The sophisticate	The striving suburbanite

Source: Beattie et al., 1993

Table 6.3 shows the range of social, behavioural and psychological variables that might be used to differentiate a target population.

Table 6.3 *Market segmentation*

Sociodemographic	Behavioural	Psychological
Location (community; neighbourhood)	Use of product/service	Self-esteem
Household size	Benefits sought	Readiness for change
Age	Level of activity	Introspection
Sex	Use of leisure	Sensation seeker
Ethnicity	Level of sexual activity	Hedonism
Nationality	Health professional utilization	Achievement orientation
Religion		Need for independence
Marital status		Societally conscious
Education		Belongers
Occupation		Need for approval
Income		Need for power
Social class		

Source: Lefebvre, 1992

The assumption behind market segmentation that the population is made up of individuals who share particular values and attitudes depending on the issue is in accord with a biographic model of health which stresses the importance of understanding individual concepts and meanings around health and moves beyond simple sociodemographic categories as a means of targeting health promotion interventions. Chapter 2 discusses the importance of research into lay meanings of health. For example, a study by Milburn (1996) describes how a healthy eating campaign for children focused entirely on its physiological benefits (living longer, not getting fat) but qualitative research with children revealed the importance they attached to the psychological benefits of not being fat and thus left out of games and "picked last".

Some social marketers segment on the basis of attitudes to health issues and disposition to change. Egger *et al.* (1993) explore the similarity between Prochaska *et al.*'s (1992) concept of an individual's readiness to change with marketing's concept of "buyer readiness" which states that at any point there are those in the population who are aware of the product, those who are informed about the product, those who are interested in buying the product, those who are motivated to buy and those who have formed an intention to buy. This awareness of the stages in behaviour change means that a target audience can be segmented according to the degree of positive attitudes to the behaviour and different messages tailored accordingly. Thus in a health promotion intervention designed to increase activity levels, the positively disposed moderately active person may get a reinforcing message, the positively disposed sedentary person might get an incentive message and the sedentary person who does not want to be more active and sees no value in it may get a confrontational message such as stressing the health risks of inactivity.

Activity

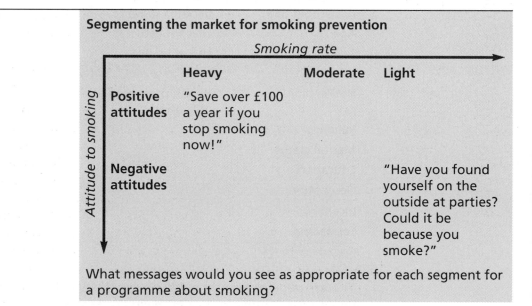

Segmenting the market for smoking prevention

What messages would you see as appropriate for each segment for a programme about smoking?

Thus smoking prevention work may be targeted to women, young people, people on a low income, Asian smokers and so on but it may also be targeted to heavy smokers or those who have tried to give up. Lefebvre (1992) describes social marketing as a "bottom up" strategy because it sets out to identify the precise interests and needs of particular groups. This is achieved through formative research such as traditional surveys, panel groups or focus groups which identify the motivations, beliefs and behaviours of the target audience. Lefebvre (1992:161) argues that "the ability to stay in close touch with consumers is too important simply to take for granted once the initial problem identification stage of programme planning is completed . . . a commitment to an on-going market research programme is vital". Pre-testing of the acceptability of the message gives the consumer some involvement and control. This is in contrast to the traditional use of the media in health promotion which tends to represent expert opinion and advice based on epidemiological data.

The selection of a target market usually follows this process:

- Epidemiological data determines which disease or condition is to be addressed.
- One or more risk factors for the disease are chosen for targeting.
- Epidemiological data is then used to identify demographic groups (including geographic and socio-economic groups) who are disproportionately represented in mortality and morbidity data.
- Qualitative research (focus groups, questionnaires, survey samples, interviews) are used to determine the attitudes, beliefs and behaviours of the target groups.
- Quantitative research is used to determine the proportion of the target group holding particular beliefs to decide if a strategy would be cost-effective.
- The selected target segments are then defined in terms of their risk behaviour and attitudes towards adopting a healthy behaviour.

Although programmes and campaigns which use marketing techniques are less prescriptive because they entail some degree of consultation, the "need" for health information is nevertheless determined through a reliance on epidemiological data. It is hard to argue that social marketing is actually an empowering process. Arnold-McCulloch and McKie (1995) suggest that the single most important contribution of social marketing to health promotion is "the skills and expertise in the appreciation of a consumer-oriented approach to campaign planning and design". The social marketer knows who the target market is and how to reach them, what are the appropriate symbols, language and values which will enhance communication with them and what beliefs and attitudes underlie their current behaviour. This knowledge helps marketers or health promoters to understand how to motivate people to change or to accept a health behaviour as important.

The message

A social marketing strategy is used to try to influence the acceptability of an idea. The idea may be quite general such as "good health"

D Department of Health guidelines on the use of educational materials concerned with nutrition suggest that materials must be appropriate to their intended users in terms of layout, content, language and level of knowledge and understanding required. They recommend consultation and pre-testing with users, particularly children. Why do you think this is particularly important with children?

or it may be a specific behaviour such as using a condom or breast feeding. A message and image has to be developed which will appeal to the target audience. The assumption of social marketers is that given the right message in the right way at the right time, people will accept and act upon it. Most texts on health promotion offer similar advice on how to "get the message across" (e.g. Egger *et al.*, 1993; Ewles and Simnett, 1995).

Make it relevant

Market research will identify the beliefs and attitudes of the target audience. The communication then needs to emphasize the similarity between the consumer and the source of the message, so that the targeted group see the issue as affecting "someone like me". The AIDS campaign used personal testimonies from a wide range of HIV-positive people to show that HIV is not confined to particular population groups and is more widespread than previously thought.

Make it credible

The acceptability of a message is influenced by the credibility of its source (Hovland and Weiss, 1951). On the one hand, people are influenced by the similarity of the image with themselves. On the other hand, when recommendations are made for change, expert knowledge is seen as most credible. The AIDS campaign decided to use doctors and public health specialists as "talking heads" in a series of advertisements in 1990 partly on this basis, but also in order to adopt a deliberately unsensational approach.

People are also more likely to adopt the attitudes of those they admire and with whom they wish to identify. Market research is used to identify opinion leaders and "significant intermediaries" for the target group. Thus many campaigns use celebrities as role models. The "Put smoking out of fashion" campaign in 1996 used fashion models to affirm they would not be photographed using cigarettes as a prop. A Health Education Authority campaign to raise awareness of testicular cancer used this well known picture of footballers Vinny Jones and Paul Gascoigne (Figure 6.1) to emphasize the need for self examination. The 1996 "Active for Life" campaign however, chose to create its own character "Daley Walker" rather than any specific role model – a pun to draw attention to physical activity but also to associate it with Daley Thompson, the well known athlete.

D What are the drawbacks of using a figurehead to lead a campaign?

The person chosen has to be acceptable to the target audience. The youth market in particular, is segmented according to music and clothes tastes and celebrities may appeal to a very narrow segment. The influence of role models may also be transitory – people may identify with the person and the message but not necessarily internalize it so that if the role model fades then the attitudes may

Figure 6.1 *Footballers Vinny Jones and Paul Gascoigne agreed to lend their support to the HEA awareness-raising campaign, promoting self-examination to detect testicular cancer. Reproduced with permission from the HEA*

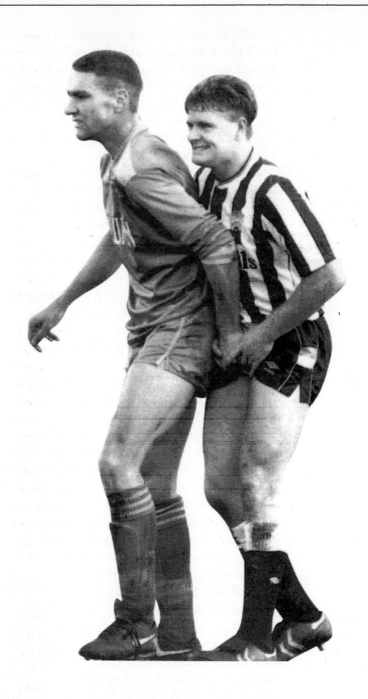

change too. The person must be credible – figureheads may end up doing the thing they are supposed to be against or vice versa. The Terrence Higgins Trust (THT) ran a series of advertisements in 1996 under the heading "The Reality Campaign". The adverts used "real" images of HIV-positive people, acknowledging the importance of an audience being able to identify with the image presented. The campaign claimed to be unusual in presenting the "reality" of sexual decision making. Most HIV/AIDS campaigns have presented a simple message – use a condom. The THT campaign acknowledged the difficulties of maintaining safer sex and challenged the assumption that HIV-positive people have an increased responsibility for safer sex (see Chapter 13 in part 3 for a further discussion of this issue).

Make it motivational

D What other motivating values are commonly linked with health messages?

A target audience needs to have reasons to adopt positive attitudes to an issue. This is where initial formative research will have highlighted likely values. In commercial marketing, a product is linked to a desired value or attribute, e.g. cars and sexual attractiveness, chocolates and escapism. When health is the product, the motivating values are often youth or energy.

Marketers state that buying a product or adopting a health message involves an exchange. The consumer pays a price, either in financial terms or in terms of time or physical or psychological effort. The price must therefore be fixed at a level which makes the benefit of the product outweigh its costs. The art of marketing according to Lefebvre (1992:167) lies in "communicating effectively the benefits of behaviour change and making the price worth it." In some instances, this may mean offering incentives to change such as a basket of fruit or leisure club voucher for quitting smoking. In health information campaigns, social marketers believe it is more effective to make explicit the costs of adopting a change in behaviour. A two-sided message may be recommended which acknowledges the benefits of a health behaviour (e.g. drinking is sociable and an aid to relaxation) but also its adverse consequences (e.g. drinking too much can lead to hangovers, driving when over the limit, unwanted sexual activity) (Hovland *et al.*, 1949). However health promoters often assume that such messages will be confusing and so simple imperatives characterize many campaigns, e.g. the "Just Say No" of recent drug prevention campaigns.

Make it seem possible

Significant changes in lifestyle may seem daunting. The individual's feelings of control and self-efficacy can be enhanced if specific actions are suggested such as calling a helpline, signing a contract with a friend to take action or specific tips on how to make a change.

Be clear, unambiguous and understood

Keep it short and simple is frequent advice. Yet trying to combine this with the attempt to attract attention often leads campaigns to adopt ambiguous messages.

R   Consider the following messages from recent campaigns. Can you identify the campaigns?

"Get the message"
"Put a Not in it"
"Slip Slap Slop"
"Kill your speed"
"A whole new ball game"
"Don't die of ignorance"

Arouse emotional involvement

Commercial advertising attracts attention in a variety of ways but dramatic images often feature prominently. When people are asked what message or image should be used for health communications they often respond that something frightening or a stern warning is needed to jolt people into action and "sit up and take notice". Health promotion campaigns have frequently used appeals to anxiety or fear. The 1986 AIDS campaign used images of tombstones carved with the word AIDS. The 1995 Drink-Driving campaign used contrasting images of young people enjoying a happy summer pub lunch with a horrific car crash. A 1994 Scottish smoking campaign used images of a young child visiting a grandparent in an oxygen tent. The use of fear in campaigns has had a varied history but strong imagery has by and large been eschewed by the lead health promotion agency in England (the HEA) since the late 1980s, following the evaluations of drug education campaigns which found the use of fear to be counterproductive (DHSS, 1987). People do not necessarily respond rationally to avoid the threat which has made them frightened and high levels of fear or repeated exposure to it can often lead to denial and disassociation from the message. On the other hand, fear may be a powerful motivator in the short term.

D

Consider the unpaid media coverage of recent health scares such as the links between eating beef and Creutzfeldt Jakob disease or between the contraceptive Pill and breast cancer. In both cases, there was a huge impact on people's behaviour immediately following the reports – beef sales dropped by 50% and large numbers of women stopped using the Pill. One year after the first reports, consumption of beef has nearly resumed its pre-BSE levels. How do you account for this?

Develop a "tangible" product which reinforces the message

A wide array of merchandise is produced to support campaigns including T-shirts, caps, bumper stickers, postcards and in the case of AIDS campaigns, condom key rings and beer mats. A very successful example of the development of a tangible product is the Red Ribbon first used by a small charity in New York in 1991 as a symbol to unite the various groups working to get the AIDS epidemic acknowledged. The Red Ribbon is recognized by 50% of the population as "something to do with AIDS" (Freeman, 1995). Its success has led to the wearing of a coloured ribbon being adopted by other groups, e.g. those working for awareness of breast cancer use a pink ribbon.

D   Why might an individual want a campaign product?

Activity

> A national campaign is being organized to raise awareness of incontinence. What could be its message?

Developing a message to promote continence is particularly difficult. It is a taboo issue which is rarely discussed in public. In addition, the term itself may not be understood. The negative effects of incontinence may be stressed such as loss of self-esteem, effects on social and sex life or the costs of sanitary protection, but this is not likely to break the taboo or encourage sufferers to seek help. Therefore the message that incontinence is both common and curable is more likely to be effective.

The place and means of promotion

Having identified the target audience and developed an appropriate message, the main channels of communication need to be identified. Channel analysis involves identifying and understanding the media habits of the target group. A variety of media can be used to reach the consumer, each of which has particular characteristics which affect message design and delivery. Electronic media such as television are considered to be, in McLuhan's (1964) well-known phrase, "hot" media which generate interest. This is in contrast to the "cooler" or more cognitive print media which can provide information. Figure 6.2 summarizes some of the main characteristics of different media and how they might be used for health promotion.

The following case study on the Sun Know How campaign illustrates how social marketing principles have become widely adopted by health promoters. Although the campaign had a clear behavioural objective and a single issue to address, extensive research was carried out. This suggested a target market of young people, particularly women. It was important to understand their attitudes to sunburn and sunbathing in order to pitch the message appropriately and to identify what value they would place on sun protection. The message was promoted through magazines but also through links with the fashion and cosmetics industries, using the channels thought to reach most young women.

Case study

Stages in the development of the Sun Know How Campaign

In 1994 the Health Education Authority led a campaign to raise awareness of skin cancer and contribute to the Health of the Nation target to halt the year-on-year increase in the incidence of skin cancer by the year 2005.

Current epidemiological knowledge suggests that malignant melanoma, which has risen from 1732 cases in 1974 to 4114 in 1989, affects younger age groups as well as older ones and is linked with exposure to short bursts of strong sunlight. Non-melanoma skin cancer is thought to be caused by cumulative exposure to the sun.

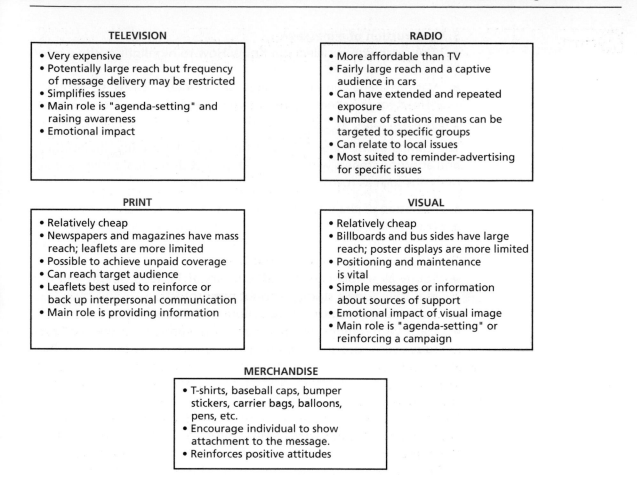

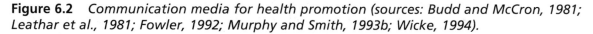

Figure 6.2 *Communication media for health promotion (sources: Budd and McCron, 1981; Leathar et al., 1981; Fowler, 1992; Murphy and Smith, 1993b; Wicke, 1994).*

1. Initial formative research

- To find out beliefs and attitudes to sunbathing and tanned skin.
- To identify demographics of target market.
- To investigate barriers to changing these attitudes and associated behaviours.

2. Formulation of campaign objectives

- To target the 13–30 age group when sunbathing starts to appeal and a tan is perceived as attractive and a boost to self-esteem.
- To highlight the risks of the sun, even in the UK.
- To reinforce existing health actions such as the use of sun screens, avoiding exposure at the hottest times of the day and restricting time spent in the sun.
- To motivate others to adopt these sun protection behaviours.
- To raise awareness that feeling and looking better isn't associated with a tan.

3. Construction of a message

- The campaign is called Sun Know How to highlight positive information objectives.
- Various behavioural messages are coined: "Dress to protect"; "Head for the shade"; "Take care not to burn".

4. Pre-testing the message

The campaign message is tested for comprehensibility, acceptability and appropriateness with the target market using qualitative research methods such as focus groups and interviews.

5. Promotion of the message

- Use various channels of communication to reach the target market, e.g. unpaid media coverage via press releases; journalist briefings especially in targeted publications.
- Lobby all scriptwriters and producers of TV soap operas and dramas to include a storyline about sun protection.
- Start Meteorological Office sunburn forecasts.
- Liaise with commercial manufacturers to promote "cover up" messages such as Sarong Know How developed with the Tie Rack outlet.

The Sun Know How campaign is illustrative of many health campaigns, its aims being to raise awareness, change attitudes and motivate people to change their behaviour. In common with other campaigns, Sun Know How:

- had a simple message or theme;
- had a defined target market ;
- used several media appropriate to the target audience and some paid advertising.

It attempted to achieve maximum publicity through a concentrated time period and with unpaid media coverage. Various merchandise were used to give the campaign a visible identity and reinforcement of the message was achieved by getting commercial companies such as Boots the Chemists and sun screen manufacturers to back the message.

A review of the Health Education Authority "Food for the Heart" campaign in 1991 suggested that campaigns could include policy and environmental objectives as well as individual behavioural ones (Velleman and Oxford, 1994). What policy or environmental objectives could be included as part of the Sun Know How mass media campaign?

Most health promoters see the design of the message as the major aspect of communication design, but deciding the place and form of promotion in which a message is disseminated are also key parts of a marketing strategy. For example, the promotion of breast feeding might be targeted at new mothers and the message disseminated at antenatal clinics. Market research shows that the target audience of women who don't wish to breast feed are young, working class mothers who are least likely to attend antenatal clinics, but who do socialize around the local shops. The campaign might therefore centre on pharmacies and grocery shops. The promotion of the message might include:

- advertising;
- personal contact;
- public relations;
- merchandising.

The following case study illustrates how a healthy eating message can be promoted in restaurants.

Case study *The Heartbeat Award*	This scheme involves issuing restaurants with an award if they meet three criteria of (i) healthy food options, (ii) a smoke free environment and (iii) good standards of food hygiene. The aim is to motivate caterers to offer healthy choices by using the incentive of the award which can be used in all publicity. It is also intended to motivate the public to eat more healthily – the award being seen as a recommendation. The Heartbeat Award scheme illustrates how social marketing principles are used in other areas of health promotion work. The scheme was intended to develop a service that consumers want. Both the caterers who receive favourable publicity and the customers who are able to choose a restaurant they know to be healthy, benefit from the exchange. In practice, evaluation has shown little consumer orientation – only 24% of the public were aware of the scheme and no one knew its title. Most establishments given the award had not changed their practice in any way in order to get it (Baxter, 1993; Murphy *et al.*, 1993). In other words, restaurants did not value the product sufficiently to make further changes. The scheme recognized the motivation for restaurants as achieving more custom but it did not achieve this. Although research had shown that people did want healthier options in restaurants, the scheme failed to achieve sufficient publicity to reach the consumer.

R	Can you think of an example of a health promotion project with which you are familiar and which you think would have benefited from social marketing. What would the benefits have been? What would be the problems or drawbacks?

So far in this chapter we have examined some of the principles of social marketing and how they are being applied to health promotion. The techniques of social marketing have wide applicability but are mostly employed when developing mass media campaigns. There are two main approaches to the study of communication.

1.   That communication is about the transmission of messages.
2.   That communication is about the meanings created and sustained through the use of various signs and symbols (Fiske, 1990).

The following section draws on different theoretical perspectives from communication and cultural studies to discuss whether marketing techniques are appropriate for promoting health through the mass media.

Health persuasion – a new panacea?

For most health promoters, communication is about transmitting a message and to do this effectively means understanding the audience, the channels and the media of communication and its effects. There are many process models of communication, all of which adopt a mechanistic and linear orientation. The American Yale–Hovland model of communication which was elaborated by McGuire (1978) is shown in Figure 6.3. It suggests that the process of mass communication entails five variables: source, message, channel, receiver and destination. As we have seen in the earlier part of this chapter, this type of model of communication underpins most media strategies. The effectiveness of the communication depends on the extent to which the source has credibility, the way the message is constructed and distributed and the receiver's receptiveness and readiness to accept the message.

Psychological models such as the Health Belief model (Becker, 1974) or the Theory of Reasoned Action (Ajzen and Fishbein, 1980)

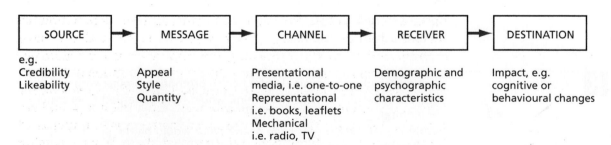

Figure 6.3   *A model of communication.*

or Ajzen's later Theory of Planned Behaviour (Ajzen, 1988) show that the simple provision of information without some modification of attitudes and beliefs, has little effect on behaviour. Nevertheless, mass media campaigns do draw on the factors highlighted in these models as influencing behaviour. Emphasis is placed on making the audience aware of the issue's relevance to them by stressing individual susceptibility through specific risk factors. The severity of the disease is also stressed but specific changes to behaviour or lifestyle are suggested to emphasize the individual's feelings of self-efficacy. Particular benefits from making a change are highlighted and barriers to change are addressed.

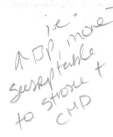

ie. ↑ BP, more susceptible to stroke + to CHD

Failure in communication is deemed to have happened when there is no impact on the receiver. On these grounds, mass media campaigns are often deemed to have failed because they cannot be shown to have contributed to any change in the population's behaviour. Tones and Tilford (1994) regard the effectiveness of the mass media as being dependent on the expected outcomes of the campaign – if these are behaviour change or a reduction in mortality or morbidity then a campaign is unlikely to be successful unless it is part of a broader programme including other complementary strategies. If the expected outcomes are raising awareness, agenda-setting or encouraging a positive attitude towards making a change, then well planned and researched campaigns can and do work.

Example

The Stanford Three Community project in the USA took three matched communities to examine the effect of different interventions on heart health. The project showed clearly how a mass media campaign in conjunction with extensive interpersonal support and advice achieved a 20% greater reduction in overall coronary heart disease (CHD) risk score compared to the community which had a mass media campaign alone (Davis, 1987).

An evaluation of the 1992 Drinkwise Wales campaign found that the campaign achieved a high awareness rating, led to increased knowledge regarding appropriate drinking levels and encouraged people to assess their own and others' drinking habits (Murphy and Smith, 1993a).

Marketers try to set realistic aims. They use the term "penetration" to indicate whether a message has reached its target and will have sophisticated methods of tracking the impact of any programme. However, there is the assumption that people are rational decision makers and once they are aware of the message, if it is relevant for them and presented in an acceptable way, they will adopt and act upon that message. The role of the social marketer is to understand the target group and therefore be able to reach them. What is missing is a recognition that socio-economic conditions present a barrier to achieving health for many people. People aren't necessarily free to choose, no matter how glossy the package.

The construction of health in advertising

Advertising has become part of our popular culture – its images and music are widely recognized and catch-phrases have entered our everyday language. Through the use of signs a message is created. For communication to take place, people need to understand these signs in the same way. According to Williamson (1984) advertising "replaces that (function) traditionally fulfilled by art or religion. It creates structures of meaning". Advertisers sell products not on the basis of their individual distinguishing features but some overall image. Volvo cars for example, are advertised in relation to their safety record. How can safety be represented in an advert? Volvo do this by using images of a family on a day out, thus appealing to and reinforcing associations between the family and values of responsibility and reliability. Signifiers (images) are used to evoke sets of meaning for the audience and which enable the communication to be understood. For example, Chapman (1993) has shown how the Marlboro cigarette advertisement of a man on a horse in open country acts as a metaphor for freedom, strength and confidence.

E **xample**

A recent series of advertisements for condoms used images of fruits (e.g. a strawberry in a woman's hand, a banana) against a bright green background. The adverts were for flavoured condoms but there was no attempt to convey a message about using a condom. Even without bodies, the adverts could be seen as being overtly sexual. The marketers had identified a young target audience who would be positively disposed to condom use and thus open to trying something new in using flavoured condoms for oral sex.

"Health" has become a value or attribute which is used to sell other products from food and clothes to cosmetics as exemplified in the huge rise of the Body Shop retail outlets. Images of youthful, active, slim (i.e. healthy) people are used to sell products whose actual use is only a small part of the message. The benefit of the product is suggested by its association with health.

D

The images associated with cornflakes have always been sunshine and the family. Sunshine makes people think of things natural and wholesome and *healthy*. The image of the family is one of nostalgia and harking back to childhood pleasures and feelings of *well-being*.
What other products can you identify which use images of health to promote the product? How is health constructed in the advertisement?

The body has become central to consumer culture (Featherstone *et al.*, 1991). The body is associated with positive attributes – looking good and feeling good. It has become a commercialized industry in which fitness, body maintenance and slimming have spawned a huge range of associated products, including videos, diet supplements, aerobics, and trainers. Yet the body has to be looked after. Here the boundaries between health and consumer culture become blurred. To look after one's body, one must be responsible and disciplined. Health thus becomes a *moral* virtue. Health and illness are located within the body which is within the control of the individual. Those who adopt unhealthy behaviour, e.g. by smoking, drinking or otherwise damaging their health, can be seen as irresponsible and even deviant. According to Bordieu (1984) consumer lifestyles can be markers of social difference. Your choice of car, food or clothes serves to make you a member of some groups and differentiate you from others. If you want to be a jetsetter, you can be seen as one by purchasing the "right" products which includes health. Being slim and fit has thus become part of lifestyle culture and is seen as a marker for success (and discipline and control).

In a similar way, health can be seen as a product which can be acquired just like a car or clothes. Health promoters believe that social marketing can help them to use advertising techniques to package "health" to various target groups. Values which are seen as desirable – youth, attractiveness, being slim, self discipline, belonging – would thus be used to "sell" health.

D

Consider the following messages which are used in health promotion campaigns. Do you regard these messages as "healthy" or "unhealthy"?

Eat well to keep in trim

Exercise to keep the body toned

Have a great social life – don't smoke

Drink sensibly to be sexy

Avoid ageing skin by protecting yourself in the sun

D   What cultural images and values could be attached to the following:

Eating vegetables
Wearing a seat belt
Installing a smoke alarm
Breast feeding
Using a condom
Using dental floss?

The dilemma for health promotion is that if it uses advertising techniques, it is most likely to be effective if it employs the images and values with which people are familiar. Those images are ones produced by a consumer culture which attempts to sell products by associating them with desirable attributes – sex, power, wealth, success, escape, fantasy, glamour, energy, fitness and youth. For health promoters, adopting marketing principles means endorsing these very stereotypes which many health promoters claim are unhealthy. Such stereotypes reinforce sexism and ageism and damage many people's self-esteem. The alternative for health promoters is to emphasize *moral* values such as responsibility, safety, conformity and social acceptance. It is precisely this difference between the worlds of commerce and health which makes the marketing of health difficult and, in the view of many, inappropriate.

The ethics of the marketplace

Marketing is predicated on the basis that individuals have the "freedom" to choose and to buy what they want and that there will be a reward or benefit from the exchange, what is termed a "voluntary and mutually beneficial exchange". The consumer gets the goods they want at an acceptable price and the manufacturer gets a profit. Yet the process is not straightforward in health promotion. The product of better public health and quality of life are, as Buchanan *et al.* (1994) point out, distant and unlikely returns. The consumer thus sees the marketing of health not as a mutually beneficial exchange but as overt persuasion. Lupton (1995) argues it is this fundamental difference in the "product" rather than any disparity in available resources between health promotion and commercial companies which makes for success in commercial marketing and makes health marketing unsuccessful.

It is through attempts to identify the benefits from an exchange that social marketers are led to construct health in ways borrowed from commercial marketing. Health must be seen as both desirable and a product, a tangible thing which it is possible to acquire.

D Can health be sold like a washing powder?

- A health message is more difficult to define than the attractions of a product and there may be different views on its benefits.
- The target audience for the health "product" are those least interested in it.
- The benefits from adopting a health message are long term as opposed to the instant gratification from using or acquiring a product.
- Health messages often involve giving up something which people value.
- The decision to adopt a health message is more complex than the relatively simple decision to purchase a product.

Marketers argue they are meeting consumers' needs by identifying what people want from a product or service. Critics argue that marketing is about the artificial creation and stimulation of wants and needs which can be met by commodities. In terms of health promotion, if a certain health behaviour is desirable, then people need to be made aware of it and why it's of value and why it would be good for them. Although people value their health as something to have, there is no actual demand for it. In fact, quite the opposite. In marketing health, health promoters are often trying to get people to give up what they perceive as desirable such as sweet things or cigarettes. The provision of health information is not meeting an unmet demand as a commercial manufacturer would argue about their product.

It could be argued that the process of surveying needs as part of social marketing is a participative strategy ensuring better targeting and meeting unmet needs. This is in contrast to the authoritarian paternalism of most health persuasion which Beattie (1991:168) describes as "employing the authority of public health expertise to re-direct the behaviour of individuals in top-down prescriptive ways". On the other hand, critics of a marketing approach to health promotion argue that it is actually a process of constructing needs according to a market model. Health promotion is constructing the individual as a health consumer who wants and needs health (Grace, 1991). This process reflects a rise in consumerism in health and social care in the last decade (Bunton *et al.*, 1995). People are deemed to be consumers with choices about what they use and what they do. They are thus responsible for their own health, preventing ill-health by "purchasing" relevant health information and services when necessary. (The extent to which this trend reflects greater accountability and participation by people in their own health care is explored further in Chapter 7 on primary health care and moves to patient choice.)

Advocates of social marketing in health promotion argue that the consumer is an active participant. People's views are sought to identify needs and then a message is developed *for* them. The lessons from these sophisticated research techniques do not, however, hide the fact that, as Lupton puts it: "social marketers seek knowledge of consumers better to influence or motivate them, not to ensure that the objectives of social marketing are considered by consumers as appropriate" (Lupton, 1995:112).

There are few simple messages when marketing health. Most media, other than print, make the communication of complex information difficult. To convey the contentiousness of much health information (e.g. the contribution of alcohol as a protective factor in Coronary Heart Disease) demands time (and therefore considerable expense) and a commitment to increasing awareness as much as changes in behaviour. Taking the example of oral health, the message to cut down on sugar is deceptively clear. But does it refer to the added sugar in drinks or cereals or the hidden sugar in most processed food? It is not possible to convey complex information about the sources of sugar or its relative risks to oral health or weight gain in an advertising campaign and so consumers are presented with insufficient information to make an informed choice about their health behaviour. Persuading people of the benefits of oral health is also difficult.

D

Which of the following images would you adopt for an oral health campaign?

- A young woman with sparkling white teeth.
- A child crying in a dentist's surgery after having a tooth filled.
- A toothbrush and pink, glossy gums with the message "Massage your gums".

Dental decay has declined with the introduction of fluoride-based toothpaste and additions to the water supply in many areas; thus the main emphasis of oral health promotion is to encourage healthy gums. The first of these images emphasizes the appearance of teeth. The second image creates anxiety and deliberately emphasizes risk. The third image encourages healthy gums but seeks to convey this message using sexual imagery. The first and third images both use people's anxiety to appear physically attractive to sell the message.

The ethics of marketing health: a checklist

- Does it promote health and make it easier for people to live healthily?
  Or can it induce guilt, raise anxiety or discomfort?
- Does it promote people's choices?
  Or does it present only partial information, not exploring its contentiousness or inconclusiveness and thereby become prescriptive?
- Is it fair?
  Or does it use scarce resources to help the better off?
- Is it a strategy which attempts to identify and meet people's needs?
  Or does it ignore particular segments of society who are harder to reach?

Conclusion

In this chapter we have seen the paradoxical relationship of health promotion with the mass media. On the one hand, health promotion is highly critical of the mass media and its influence. Considerable efforts are devoted to campaigning against tobacco advertising on the grounds that it encourages new smokers. Many of the risk factors for disease – sedentary lifestyle, unhealthy eating, unprotected sex – are shaped by a consumer culture which promotes unhealthy products such as junk food and confectionery and presents risky behaviours such as excessive alcohol intake or fast and reckless driving as acceptable. Health promoters criticize how the public perception of health issues is generally related to illness rather than positive health due to the reporting of hospital-based medicine and technological wizardry (Naidoo and Wills, 1994).

On the other hand, health promotion endeavours to use marketing techniques (which it sees as effective) to promote health. In so doing, it is in danger of reinforcing some of those negative attributes so readily seen in the marketing of commodities. The argument presented in this chapter is that although a social marketing approach to health promotion may be an effective way of targeting information and changing attitudes and behaviour, it still tends to be professionally and epidemiologically driven. In particular, there may be a conflict between marketing's concept of the individual as a consumer and health promotion's concept of individuals as participating and autonomous citizens. Health promoters swayed by the idea that marketing techniques may be more equitable and empowering for target groups need also to weigh up the ethics of attempts to persuade people that health is something they need and want.

D Why do you think marketing tactics and media campaigns are so popular in health promotion?

The simple answer must be that a mass media campaign is visible. Health promoters can be seen to be doing something about the nation's health. Campaigns are often specified in health promotion contracts. The Department of Health document "First Steps for the NHS" specifies that District Health Authority contracts and provider business plans should include mounting campaigns to coincide with National No Smoking Day, Drinkwise Day and other local and national initiatives (Department of Health, 1992).

In Chapter 5 we saw how targeting health promotion needs to be treated with some caution. If targeting is adopted, then marketing does have certain lessons for health promotion. The practice of understanding the client group through careful and systematic research rather than professional assumptions is important. Equally important is to recognize the diversity of health beliefs and to move beyond simple socio-demographic categories for targeting. Information and messages can be tailored to particular audiences and do not need to follow the common sense assumption that "short and simple" is best. Marketing thus provides useful techniques and skills for health promotion. However, it does have major limitations as a health promotion strategy. The role of poverty as the principal determinant of ill-health in our society needs to be recognized. Marketing's use of the concepts of both "individual" and "health" constructs health as a personal choice.

Activity

Draw up a marketing strategy for one of the following:

Breast feeding	Use of medicines
Sensible drinking	Weight control
Home safety	Stress reduction

You will need to decide:

■   The market or target audience.

- The market segment (if any).
- The marketing mix, i.e.
  - □ the product and its key characteristics;
  - □ the price and how important it is for the audience;
  - □ the place (where the message would be promoted);
  - □ the promotion (how the message is to be presented).

How easy or difficult did you find this exercise?
What can you learn from this for your own work and how you present information?

Further discussion

- Are marketing and health promotion fundamentally compatible or incompatible?
- How does marketing construct health as a personal choice?
- Four key principles of health promotion are:
  - □ equity
  - □ collaboration
  - □ participation
  - □ empowerment.

  How do these relate to the concept of marketing?

Recommended reading

- Egger G, Donovan R and Spark R (1993) *Health and the media: principles and practice for health promotion*, Sydney, McGraw Hill.

  A comprehensive and accessible guide to using different media for health promotion. Combines practical advice, examples (mostly from Australia) and some underpinning theory.

- Fiske J (1990) *Introduction to communication studies*, London, Routledge.

  A clear introduction to communication analysis and the cultural meanings of different media communications.

- A series of articles discussing the arguments for and against the application of marketing techniques to health promotion:

  Hastings GB and Haywood AJ (1991) Social marketing and communication in health promotion, *Health Promotion International*, 6(2), 135–45.

  Buchanan DR, Reddy S and Hossain Z (1994) "Social marketing: a critical response", *Health Promotion International*, 9(1), 49–57.

  Hastings GB and Haywood AJ (1994) "Social marketing: a critical response" *Health Promotion International*, 9(1), 59–63.

- Lefebvre RC (1992) "Social marketing and health promotion" in Bunton R and Macdonald G (eds) *Health promotion: Disciplines and Diversity*, London, Routledge.
  A useful introduction to the value of social marketing which is seen as a problem-solving technique enabling careful planning and accurate targeting.

- Tones K and Tilford S (1994) *Health Education: Effectiveness, efficiency and equity*, London, Chapman Hall.
  Summarizes the main studies on the effectiveness of health promotion using the media and includes a section on social marketing.

References

Ajzen I (1988) *Attitudes, personality and behaviour*, Buckingham, Open University Press.

Ajzen I and Fishbein M (1980) *Understanding attitudes and predicting behaviour*, Englewood Cliffs, N.J., Prentice Hall.

Arnold-McCulloch R and McKie L (1995) "The potential application of social marketing techniques in health promotion", *Journal of Institute of Health Education*, **32**(4), 120–25.

Baxter P (1993) *Heartbeat Award Monitoring Report*, London, Health Education Authority.

Beattie A (1991) "Knowledge and control: a test case for social policy and social theory", in Gabe J, Calnan M and Bury M (eds) *Sociology of the Health Service*, London, Routledge.

Beattie A, Gott M, Jones L and Sidell M (eds) (1993) *Health and Wellbeing: A Reader*, Basingstoke, Macmillan/Open University.

Becker MH (1974) *The health belief model and personal health behaviour*, Health Education Monographs, **2**, 324–508.

Bordieu P (1984) *Distinction: a social critique of the judgement of taste*, London, Routledge.

Buchanan DR, Reddy S and Hossain Z (1994) "Social marketing: a critical appraisal", *Health Promotion International*, **9**(1), 49–57.

Budd J and McCron R (1981) "Health Education and the mass media: past, present and future", in Leathar DS, Davies JK and Hastings G (eds) *Health Education and the Media*, Oxford, Pergamon.

Bunton R, Nettleton S and Burrows R (1995) *Sociology of Health Promotion*, London, Routledge.

Chapman S (1993) "Myth in cigarette advertising and health promotion", in Beattie A (ed.) *Health and Wellbeing: a reader*, Basingstoke, Macmillan.

Department of Health (1992) *The Health of the Nation*, London, HMSO.

DHSS (1987) *Anti heroin campaign: Stage Five Research evaluation*, London, DHSS.

Davis AM (1987) "Heart Health Campaigns", *Health Education Journal*, **39**, 74–79.

Downie RS, Fyfe C and Tannahill A (1990) *Health Promotion: Models and Values*, Oxford, Oxford Medical Publications.

Egger G, Donovan R and Spark R (1993) *Health and the media: principles and practice for health promotion*, Sydney, McGraw Hill.

Ewles L and Simnett I (1995) *Promoting health: a practical guide*, London, Scutari.

Featherstone M, Hepworth M and Turner BS (eds) (1991) *The Body: social process and cultural theory*, London, Sage.

Fiske J (1990) *Introduction to Communication Studies*, London, Routledge.

Flora A and Lefebvre RC (1988) "Social marketing and public health interventions", *Health Education Quarterly*, **15**(3), 299–315.

Fowler G (1992) "Health education in general practice: the use of leaflets", *Health Education Journal*, **44**(3), 149–50.

Freeman D (1995) *World AIDS Day Evaluation Report*, London, Health Education Authority.

Grace VM (1991) "The marketing of empowerment and the construction of the health consumer: a critique of health promotion", *International Journal of Health Services*, **21**(2), 329–43.

Hastings G and Haywood A (1991) "Social marketing and communication in health promotion", *Health Promotion International*, **6**(2), 135–45.

Hovland CI and Weiss W (1951) "The influence of source credibility on communication effectiveness", *Public Opinion Quarterly*, **15**, 635–50.

Hovland CI, Lumsdaine AA and Sheffield FD (1949) *Experiments on mass communication*, Princeton N.J., Princeton University Press.

Kotler P and Zaltman G (1971) "An approach to planned social change", *Journal of Marketing*, **35**, 3–12.

Leathar DS, Hastings GB and Davies JK (eds) (1981) *Health Education and the Media*, vol. 1, Oxford, Pergamon Press.

Lefebvre RC (1992) "Social marketing and health promotion", in Bunton R and Macdonald G (eds) *Health promotion: Disciplines and Diversity*, London, Routledge.

Lupton D (1995) *The Imperative of health*, London, Sage.

McGuire WJ (1978) *Evaluating advertising: a bibliography of the communication process*, Advertising Research Foundation.

McLuhan M (1964) *Understanding Media*, London, Routledge Kegan Paul.

Milburn K (1996) "The importance of lay theorising for health promotion research and practice", *Health Promotion International*, **11**, 141–47.

Murphy S and Smith C (1993a) "Drinkwise Wales 1992: an evaluation of the campaign", *Health Education Journal*, **512**, 227–30.

Murphy S and Smith C (1993b) "Crutches, confetti or useful tools: professional's view on the use of health education leaflets", *Health Education Research*, **8**(2), 205–15.

Murphy S, Powell C and Smith C (1993) "A formative evaluation of the Welsh Heartbeat Award Scheme", *Nutrition and Health*, 317–27.

Naidoo J and Wills J (1994) *Health Promotion: Foundations for Practice*, London, Baillière Tindall.

Prochaska J, DiClemente C and Norcross JC (1992) "In search of how people change", *American Psychologist*, **47**, 1102–14.

Tones K and Tilford S (1994) *Health Education: effectiveness, efficiency and equity*, London, Chapman Hall.

Velleman G and Oxford L (1994) "Issues in implementing a national HEA campaign at local level", *Health Education Journal*, **53**, 182–93.

Wicke DM (1994) "Effectiveness of waiting room noticeboards as a vehicle for health education", *Family Practice*, **11**(3), 292–95.

Williams G (1985) "Health Promotion – caring concern or slick salesmanship", *Journal of the Institute of Health Education*, **23**(1), 423–30.

Williamson J (1984) *Decoding advertisements*, London, Marion Boyars.

7 *Health promotion in a primary care led NHS*

Key points

- How recent changes in the NHS affect health promotion within primary healthcare (PHC).
- Health promotion in the PHC setting – the arguments for and against.
- Effectiveness of health promotion in PHC – differences in perspective.
- Opportunistic health promotion within PHC.
- Planned health promotion and screening within PHC.
- Competing views of what health promotion should be within PHC: medical model versus Health for All model.

Overview

Recent reforms and changes in funding have sought to implement a "primary healthcare led NHS". The aim is that decision taking about purchasing and providing healthcare should be taken by GPs and primary healthcare teams working closely with patients (NHS Executive, 1995). The role and importance of primary healthcare has been stressed. Primary healthcare (PHC), or first level healthcare delivered in community settings, is uniquely accessible and acceptable to the vast majority of the population. PHC has therefore immense potential to deliver not only first level care and treatment, but also prevention and health promotion. Whilst these changes provide new opportunities for health promotion, there are also constraints and problematic features. The dilemmas and challenges posed for health promotion located within a PHC setting are the focus of this chapter.

First, the policy context in which health promotion within PHC has become prioritized is outlined. The economic climate has placed an emphasis on "value for money" and led to a focus on proven effectiveness. The requirement for evidence-based practice within the NHS applies to health promotion activities as well as to treatment protocols. This has led to increased interest in monitoring health promotion delivery within PHC settings. PHC practitioners are now involved in a range of health promotion activities including chronic disease and general population screening and opportunistic advice. The opportunities this raises for health promotion are discussed together with a critique which examines the problems of delivering health promotion within PHC.

In addition to the many practical problems of fitting health promotion into PHC which is already being stretched to the limit, there are problems of orientation or perspective. The strengths of PHC lie in its accessible and high quality medical services. Trying to shift PHC to a broader Health for All (HFA) perspective advocated by the World Health Organization

(WHO) is a huge and daunting task which risks failure. An alternative perspective would be to not prioritize the PHC setting through funding arrangements, but to broaden out the funding and responsibility for health promotion.

Introduction

Primary healthcare (PHC) was the focus of the World Health Organization's (WHO) conference at Alma Ata in 1978. The WHO declaration, signed by 134 participating countries, stated that PHC was the key to achieving Health for All by the year 2000 (HFA 2000).

> "Primary health care is essential health care based on practical, scientifically sound and socially acceptable methods and technology made universally accessible to individuals and families in the community through their full participation and at a cost that the community and country can afford in the spirit of self-reliance and determination"
>
> (WHO, 1978:vi).

PHC was envisioned as the means by which healthcare services could become more accessible and appropriate to populations, and the WHO advocated a shift of resources from hospital provision to community health provision. But the WHO declaration went further than this. Three central pillars to PHC were identified:

- **Participation** – people have the right to determine actively the planning and delivery of health services.
- **Intersectoral collaboration** – health is determined by many social, environmental and economic factors which go beyond the remit of health service provision. In order to promote health, different sectors, e.g. education, environmental services, housing, income support, transport, agriculture and social welfare need to collaborate with each other.
- **Equity** – existing inequalities in health need to be reduced through the provision of appropriate services which reach everybody. This entails a fairer allocation of health resources.

Underlying these principles is a concept of holistic positive health including social, environmental, mental, emotional and physical dimensions.

Although the UK was a signatory member of the Alma Ata conference, it could be argued that recent developments in PHC have not been undertaken with these principles in mind. Instead, recent reforms of the NHS have been driven by market principles of competition and funding and the increase of managerial power at the expense of professional or client power (Williams *et al.*, 1993). Although recent NHS reforms, in particular GP fundholding (whereby GPs become budget holders who buy in services for their patients), have sought to direct resources into primary care, the concept of PHC remains traditional, centred on medical treatment of individuals. Resources for health promotion are increasingly channelled via GPs, through first the 1993 GP contract bandings payments and then the 1996 payment regulations for health promotion activities. The NHS is acknowledged as the lead agency in promoting health but there is no infrastructure or resourcing to make intersectoral collaboration a reality.

Health promotion within PHC

Recent NHS reforms set the scene for health promotion delivery in PHC settings. Key features of the reforms are given in Table 7.1.

The health market

The purchaser/provider split was introduced, with a distinction between commissioning health authorities which purchase services

Table 7.1 *Recent NHS Reforms and their impact on health promotion*

1987 "Promoting Better Health" This introduced new contracts for doctors and dentists which included incentive payments for health checks and achieving target levels of vaccination, immunization and screening. Health promotion and disease prevention are highlighted as key objectives. Other principles include raising standards of care and providing information and choice for patients.

1989 "Working for Patients" This aimed to address problems in management and financing within the NHS, to increase the efficiency with which resources are used, and to enable services to be more responsive to users. The document introduced GP budget-holding and a new GP contract which provided financial incentives for health clinics in addition to health checks, vaccination and immunization. The document also sought to strengthen management at all levels including the more effective management of clinical activity and resource allocation.

Care in the Community Act 1990 led to more people requiring long-term care being moved from institutions into the community. Demographic changes mean that an increasing percentage of the population is elderly or very elderly, with associated increased healthcare needs. Whilst the move to community care is welcomed as increasing client autonomy, there is little provision or resourcing for the higher levels of demand being made on community based staff. There are also fears that carers are being left to cope on their own, without support or advice.

1990 NHS Reforms These wide-ranging reforms sought to introduce the principles of market competition and public accountability within the NHS. Health promotion continues to be encouraged through financial remuneration as a discrete activity carried out in PHC settings under the direction of GPs. Two key features of these reforms are the health market and accountability.

to meet the needs of their local populations, and provider trusts which provide healthcare services. The principle of market place competition between competing service providers was endorsed as a means of delivering cost-effective service provision. Critics argue that this philosophy is inappropriate for healthcare and that a climate of competition contradicts and impedes the process of teamwork and inter-agency collaboration.

GP fundholding was extended until, by 1997, around half the population are covered by fundholding arrangements. This enabled GPs to purchase a range of services for their patients and to employ practitioners, usually practice nurses, who may be delegated to undertake health promotion activities. The 1996 Audit Commission Report questioned the effectiveness of fundholding as a means of health service delivery. The new Labour government is likely to suspend or even end fundholding in favour of locality commissioning.

Accountability

The Patient's Charter spelled out the rights of patients to high quality services. The principle used is that of consumerism. Whilst consumer groups welcomed this initiative, many practitioners, especially GPs, feel it exposes them to unreasonable demands and the fear of litigation. There were also fears that patients may become "doctor shoppers".

Contract arrangements

The 1990 GP contract which funded health promotion clinics was replaced by the 1993 revised GP contract which introduced three banding levels for health promotion activity. The focus of this activity was on risk factor assessment and management, especially in relation to coronary heart disease and stroke. Chronic disease management clinics for asthma and diabetes were also funded. Most of this activity was delegated by GPs to their practice nurses. The effectiveness of such activity has been questioned, and there have been many complaints about the amount of paperwork involved. This has led to the 1996 revised contract arrangements.

The new 1996 health promotion arrangements are based on the following principles (Hasler, 1994):

- GPs will be able to choose whether to adopt opportunistic or more formal health promotion activities.
- Monitoring will be professionally led.
- Bureaucracy will be kept to a minimum.
- GPs will not be encouraged to carry out activities which are not backed by scientific evidence.

The 1996 revised GP contract states that GPs must submit proposed health promotion activities for approval by a local Health Promotion

Committee (led by Local Medical Committees with GP representatives), and later in the year confirm such activities have been undertaken (or state what alternatives have been adopted and why). It is estimated that the average payment to GPs will be £2165 per annum or £1.17 per patient (1996 prices).

Why deliver health promotion within PHC?

> **D** Contractual arrangements for the delivery of health promotion within PHC have changed three times since 1990. What factors could account for such rapid change?

At first sight, delivering health promotion within PHC has many advantages. The primary healthcare team (PHCT) has unique access to the whole population. Over 97% of the poplation is registered with a GP and over 70% of patients consult their GP at least once a year (Office of Health Economics, 1994). Almost all of the registered population will visit their GP during a five-year period (Royal College of General Practitioners, 1986). Doctors and nurses are seen as highly credible sources of information, and advice on health matters from them is both expected and accepted.

PHC practitioners already operate as teams, although the size and nature of these teams varies considerably. A core team of GP, practice nurse, practice manager and administrative staff is often complemented by a broader team including community-based nurses, professions allied to medicine (e.g. dietitians, speech therapists, chiropodists, physiotherapists, counsellors) and, more rarely, other welfare workers such as social workers. Members of the primary healthcare team (PHCT) provide continuity of service together with easy access, which is valued by clients. PHC practitioners usually see clients on a one-to-one basis which allows information and advice to be individually tailored.

The 1993 banding payment structure required practices to complete standard forms recording risk factor assessment for their registered population. The intention was to create a comprehensive database of the practice population which could be used to identify priorities and as a base-line for monitoring. However, the arrangements were criticized for being too centralized and not allowing local needs to influence the data collected, and as a bureaucratic exercise in information collection for its own sake.

The potential of the data collection requirements was not maximized. Data collection could have provided the opportunity for the practice population to be viewed as a socially consituted group and would have allowed links to be made between health status and social influences. Instead the practice population was seen as a collection of individuals. Depending on how this data was collected and used, it also provided opportunities for the PHCT to shift their way of working from a medically dominated, expert led practice to a more genuinely collaborative and participatory practice.

Activity

> Some practices included open-ended questions which people could use to identify their own health needs. Some practices took the opportunity to routinely record housing, income or occupational status on patient records. What other aspects can you identify which would maximize the potential of the data collection exercise to promote health in the broadest sense?

As the NHS is encouraged to move towards evidence-based practice, proponents of health promotion claim that health promotion in PHC settings is an effective use of resources, using recent research studies to support their claims (MacPherson, 1994; Doyle and Thomas, 1996). Sceptics argue that such activities are not effective. The issue of effectiveness is discussed in greater detail later on p. 146.

Arguments against health promotion within PHC

Is health promotion in PHC settings appropriate and relevant?

The implications of delivering health promotion through PHC have been viewed in a less positive light by many commentators. GPs and others interpreted the 1993 contractual requirement to collect data on risk factors as an extension of managerialism and an attack on professional expertise (Taylor and Bloor, 1994; Yen, 1995). Many practitioners complained that such information was more useful for managers than clinicians, and that the collection of such information intrudes on the practitioner/client relationship.

The time taken to collect this data meant less time to actually deliver health information or advice. With time at such a premium within the PHC setting, many practitioners questioned whether data collection represents the best use of scarce resources. The reliability of data collected has also been disputed. For example, there were no guidelines given for measuring hypertension, with the result that different practices used different threshold values. This meant comparisons between different practices were not always valid. It was partly the strength of these arguments which led to an agreement in 1996 to change the health promotion funding arrangements for general practice.

The banding structure was seen as inflexible and incapable of responding to specific health needs of locally registered populations. The banding structure prioritized risk factors for coronary heart disease (CHD) and stroke, and recognized the need for chronic disease management clinics. Local knowledge may suggest other diseases or conditions may be more relevant to the local population, but there was no remuneration for health promotion activity directed towards anything other than CHD and stroke.

D

CHD is the major cause of premature death in Britain. Does this justify it being the major condition to be screened for in all general practices? What would be your view if the practice was:

■ located in an inner city area with a high proportion of homeless and temporarily housed young families?

■ located in an area with a high proportion of families from Black and minority ethnic communities?

■ located in a rural area characterized by isolation, poor public transport, and few social networks?

■ located in a residential area, close to a university, with a high proportion of students?

There is a constant tension for practitioners between responding to demands for the treatment of symptoms and ill-health on the one hand, and pressures to be pro-active in preventing ill-health or promoting health on the other. Many GPs would argue that their particular expertise is in diagnosis and treatment, not health promotion, and are uncomfortable with a role as health promoters despite the extra payments which accompany this.

R

Consider the following comments from GPs. If you were seeking to enhance health promotion in PHC, how would you respond?

"I didn't come into general practice in order to tell people how they should live their lives."

"Patients don't need my advice about healthy lifestyles."

"General practice is a demand led service. I feel uncomfortable foisting health checks and advice on patients who have come to me because they are ill."

"I am a health professional, not an undercover police officer collecting information for the government."

Most health promotion in PHC is delegated by GPs to practice nurses. Since 1988 the number of full-time equivalent practice nurses has trebled (Atkin and Hirst, 1994). The banding structure marked health promotion as a separate "add-on" activity rather than an activity integral to all consultations. It remains to be seen whether or not the revised 1996 contract will lead to the integration of health promotion within PHC and what kind of health promotion activities will be proposed by GPs.

Are PHC team members adequately trained and motivated to carry out health promotion activities?

Whilst practice and community nurses may feel more confident and committed to health promotion as part of their job, work priorities all too often lie elsewhere. Health promotion is often at the bottom of the list, viewed as a "luxury extra" to be fitted in if time allows. Research studies have shown that "lack of time" is frequently cited as a reason for not undertaking more health promotion (Kaufman, 1990; Coronary Prevention Group, 1993).

The issue of whether members of the PHCT have sufficient training in health promotion to ensure effective delivery of interventions has been flagged up in many studies (e.g. Doyle and Thomas, 1996). There is debate about what constitutes the necessary training and skills to promote health in PHC. Many studies identify good communication and interpersonal skills, teamwork skills and confidence in the health promotion role. These issues have already been discussed in Chapter 1. Teamwork is often cited as an important aspect of effective delivery of health promotion in PHC. Yet one study found little evidence of collaboration – only 27% of GPs and district nurses with patients in common, and 11% of GPs and health visitors (Gregson *et al.*, 1992), communicated about their shared patients.

Knowledge and information about appropriate lifestyle changes may also be lacking. A literature review of nutrition interventions in primary healthcare states that problems included ". . . insufficient nutritional knowledge and dietary counselling skills . . ." (Coronary Prevention Group, 1993).

PHCT members may not feel confident about their health promotion role. Recent policies have meant that, far from encouraging and building on the opportunities for teamwork within the PHCT, most practices siphon off health promotion as a specific activity undertaken by practice nurses. The huge rise in numbers of practice nurses has not been matched by an increase in training opportunities. As employees of GPs, practice nurses are reliant on individual GPs' enthusiasm to fund their training. Most practice nurses work part-time, so opportunities for training are limited. Most also come from a clinical rather than a community background. As a result, practice nurses are likely to have a narrow view of health promotion and their role as a health promoter. One recent study found that most practice nurses perceive themselves as having an educational role but few agreed with the statement that health promotion should include meeting people to work together to change health policy (Wilson Barnett and Macleod Clark, 1993). In this same study, only 2% suggested that they adopted a social model of health. Most practice nurses rely on leaflets and individual advice, whilst the potential for group work and targeting those in need is neglected.

The "stages of change" approach to behaviour change (Prochaska and DiClemente, 1984) has received recent popularity and been the focus of a training programme for PHCT members supported by the HEA. See Figure 7.1 for a summary of this model.

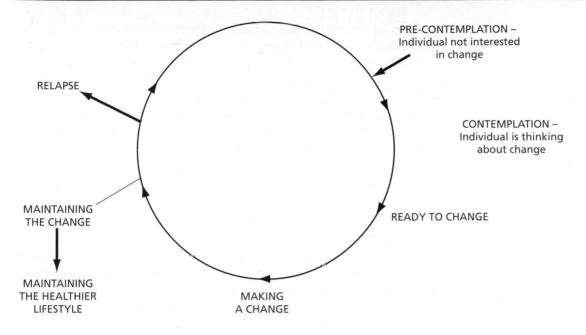

Figure 7.1   *Stages of Change Model (Prochaska and DiClemente; from Naidoo and Wills, 1994).*

This approach emphasizes that education and advice need to be tailored towards individuals and their readiness to receive and act upon behaviour change messages. It suggests that before embarking on health education, a "diagnosis" should be undertaken – to find out whether an individual is committed to lifestyle changes and sees change as realistic in their circumstances. The "stages of change" model is useful in that it helps PHCT members direct their energies to where they will be most effective. It is, however, quite limited in scope, in that it equates health promotion with individual advice, information or empowerment, and does not look beyond to community development or participation.

D   In what ways could the adoption of the "stages of change" model be said to reinforce inequalities in health?

Research suggests that practice nurses find it easiest, and most rewarding, to target those people who are willing and able to change their lifestyles, such as middle class people, rather than those who stand to benefit most from such changes (Daykin *et al.*, 1995).

The rate of organizational and policy change has led to increased workloads and stress for PHC practitioners. In the midst of ongoing change and more stringent requirements concerning accountability, the enthusiasm and goodwill necessary to implement further changes to promote health in the the PHC setting is lacking (Kaufman, 1990). In particular, many practitioners have felt they were being asked to "pick up the pieces" in PHC, whilst the government is failing in its duty to support this work with appropriate policies (Orme and Wright, 1996; Daykin and Naidoo, 1997).

Is health promotion in PHC effective?

A major problem with gaining commitment to health promotion in PHC is uncertainty and doubt about the effectiveness of health promotion.

E xample	Two major studies, widely reported in the medical press, found only modest changes in patients' risk factor status despite intensive screening and health education activity by practice nurses (Family Heart Study Group, 1994; OXCHECK Study Group, 1994, 1995). The FHSG study found a 16% reduction in coronary risk score and a 4% reduction in smoking rate, which if maintained long-term would lead to a 12% reduction in the risk of coronary events. However, the practice nurse activity (screening and advice) was very intensive and not thought to be generally replicable.
The Family Heart Study Group (FHSG) and OXCHECK research studies into effectiveness of health promotion in PHC	The OXCHECK study investigated the effect of one-hour practice nurse/patient sessions which focused on screening and counselling. Smoking cessation results were poor, but there was improved management by patients with hypertension and high cholesterol levels. (Source: FHSG, 1994; OXCHECK, 1994, 1995.)

Critics have argued that these findings demonstrate that to pursue health promotion in PHC is to ignore the call to base practice on evidence of effectiveness. However, more sympathetic commentators have argued that the findings are sufficiently positive to support further work in this area. Doyle and Thomas (1996:5) found ". . . different reactions to these studies from public health and primary care staff. Directors of Public Health noted potentially respectable health-gain at a population level . . . while primary care commentators saw the results as vindication of their argument for abandoning such methods of health promotion."

Recent research into the cost-effectiveness of the Family Heart Study Group and OXCHECK Study Group interventions concluded that "the more intensive British family heart study intervention was more effective but less cost effective than the OXCHECK intervention" and that "The cost effectiveness of these (interventions) crucially depends on the assumed duration of the risk reduction, which must persist for at least five years for either programme to be viewed as cost effective" (Wonderling *et al.*, 1996:1278).

At present, it would seem that there is sufficient evidence to persuade those already predisposed towards health promotion to continue their efforts, but not enough to persuade sceptics. There is an urgent need to carry out further research to determine the long-term effectiveness of health promotion interventions within PHC.

Differences in perspective

There is a need for a "paradigm shift" or shift in how health and health promotion are conceptualized within PHC. Health is not just about reducing morbidity and mortality, it is also about supporting people in adverse circumstances and maximizing everyone's potential for health. For example, improving quality of life is a valid health promotion goal. Research studies support the role of health promotion in enhancing the quality of life of people with medical conditions (Cupples *et al.*, 1996). The problem lies in the different epistemological (knowledge) and practice basis for health promotion and PHC. These differences are summarized in Table 7.2.

Table 7.2 *The different epistemological and practice basis for health promotion and primary healthcare*

Health promotion – core principles	Health promotion in PHC
Population approach	Individual practitioner/patient relationship
Seeks to empower people	A set of activities "bolted on" to clinical practice directed towards patients
Intersectoral work is encouraged	Health promotion usually isolated from clinical practice and the responsibility of practice nurses
Seeks to redress inequalities	May reinforce inequalities by addressing needs of the most accessible patients
Active participation is encouraged	Patient compliance valued above participation
Evaluation in terms of processes and outcomes	Evaluation in terms of reduced morbidity and mortality
Focus on holistic health	Focus on medical conditions

Opportunistic and planned health promotion

There are two models of promoting health in PHC settings: opportunistic and planned activities. Opportunistic health promotion is unplanned but fitted into consultations or clinics when appropriate. Planned health promotion is prepared in advance, allowing more time to set objectives and think about how to evaluate the activity. Health promotion or screening clinics are an example of planned health promotion. The dilemmas surrounding each model of practice is discussed in further detail below.

Opportunistic health promotion

Activity

> What (if any) kind of opportunistic health promotion would be appropriate for the following?
> What kind of considerations would affect whether or not you gave opportunistic health advice and information?
>
> - A mother of two attending a family planning clinic for a pill check.
> - A middle-aged woman attending surgery for a repeat prescription of anti-depressants.
> - An older man attending the treatment room for leg ulcer dressing.
> - A young mother attending emergency surgery with her two year old who has been scalded by hot water.

The benefits of opportunistic health promotion include cheapness, minimum disruption to established work routines and adaptability to individual circumstances. An early study which showed that five-minutes of advice about smoking cessation given opportunistically by GPs to patients resulted in a 5% cessation rate after one year (Russell *et al.*, 1979) was influential in winning converts to opportunistic health promotion. More recent research supports the view that opportunistic health promotion is more effective than the planned clinic approach (Wilson *et al.*, 1992; Doyle and Thomas, 1996). However, inadequate training means that there are lost opportunities too, e.g. practice nurses rarely raise sexual health issues with clients.

The problems of opportunistic health promotion – its *ad hoc* nature, a lack of clear objectives and difficulty in monitoring its effectiveness – have led policy makers and many practitioners to prefer planned health promotion. There are also ethical concerns. For example, carrying out opportunistic health checks might raise the issue of whether informed consent was given for this procedure, since the patient did not consult for the purpose of a health check (Doxiadis, 1987).

Planned health promotion and screening

Health promotion clinics

Planned health promotion includes risk factor screening and health promotion clinics such as asthma management or well person checks, when people are invited to attend PHC surgeries or clinics for specific, predetermined preventive healthcare measures. PHC practitioners may "bolt on" opportunistic health education or advice in planned clinic settings. For example, someone attending an asthma management clinic may be given advice on diet or exercise.

Arguments for health promotion clinics include efficiency, better targeting and possible spin-offs such as increased networking and social support. Arguments against include concerns with equity in the light of research which reports that preventive clinic provision is used most by middle class people who enjoy better health (Waller *et al.*, 1990; Griffiths *et al.*, 1994) as well as concerns about the effectiveness of such activity.

Community profiling

Community profiling, when the practice investigates local perceptions of health needs and epidemiological data to build a picture of local priorities and resources, provides another example of planned health promotion, albeit non-funded. Health visitors and community workers are trained in community profiling skills, and may have already undertaken such a profile. Community profiles can aid the transition from focusing on individual patients to practice populations.

Screening

Risk factor screening clinics provide a useful case study of planned health promotion. Many different kinds of screening clinics have been established and evaluated, ranging from well woman to coronary heart disease risk factors to child health.

R What is your definition of screening?

One definition of screening, accepted by the WHO Regional Committee for Europe, is:

> "the presumptive identification of a recognised disease or defect by the application of tests, examinations and other procedures which can be applied rapidly. Screening tests sort out apparently well persons who probably have a disease from those who probably do not. A screening test is not intended to be diagnostic"
>
> (Commission on Chronic Illness, 1957).

There are other kinds of screening in use today. We can categorize screening into four different types:

1. Detection of specific diseases before symptoms appear, e.g. breast and cervical cancer screening, coronary heart disease screening.
2. Anonymous screening used to detect trends in public health but not linked to treatment, e.g. anonymous HIV screening of pregnant women.
3. Health screening not linked to any particular disease, but looking at lifestyles in general, e.g. well woman clinics.
4. Genetic screening investigating inheritable factors in order to assist parenting decisions, e.g. sickle cell screening.

D What screening might take place in the PHC setting? What factors would need to be taken into account to determine good practice?

Examples of screening in PHC settings include practice nurses carrying out cervical smear tests and health visitors doing child development testing at a child health clinic. The acceptability of screening depends on a number of factors, such as who carries out the test, where it takes place, how uncomfortable or invasive the test is, whether a standard protocol is followed, how long it takes for the results, and how results are given.

E xample

Cervical cancer screening

The 1990 GP contract included financial incentives for practices to achieve targets of 80% uptake of cervical screening amongst the relevant practice population. This encouraged the establishment of the call/recall system in which eligible women are identified from practice records and invited to attend for a smear. The introduction of targets created fears that patients might be excluded from practice lists if they refused screening tests, or might be subjected to pressure to take the test if the target was almost within reach.

Concerns have been voiced that, for some women, pressure to accept screening for reasons not connected to their own health constitutes a negative health experience overall. All health interventions should have clear benefits which outweigh the disbenefits or costs. Raising expectations of a screening programme when there are insufficient resources allocated to provide a high quality service is unethical.

Stigma surrounding risk factors also affects the acceptability of screening. For example, the link between multiple sexual partners and cervical cancer is potentially stigmatizing, and women may avoid screening in order to avoid being stigmatized if they test positive. Ignorance and fear of the condition being screened for are a further problem in acceptability. Some people are so scared by the thought of cancer that they refuse cancer screening tests.

(Chapter 11 looks further at this issue.)

E xample

Child health screening

The purpose of child health surveillance is traditionally the identification of problems. But the latest edition of "Health for all Children" from the Joint Working Party on child health surveillance (Hall, 1996) uses the term "child health promotion". Child health checks used to be organized around ensuring children performed specific tasks competently, the purpose of which was to identify developmental problems. This approach is changing. The effectiveness of routine screening is questionable, but health visitors are keen to retain a core surveillance programme.

"The promotion of child health requires a shift in the relationship between parents, children and health professionals to one of partnership rather than supervision in which parents are empowered to make use of services and expertise according to their needs" (Hall, 1996:9).

Research into pilot projects has identified the following good practice criteria (Larner *et al.*, 1992):

- Services are broad spectrum and comprehensive, crossing traditional professional boundaries and are coherent and easy to use.
- Both the structure and the individual staff are flexible in their ability to respond to unexpected demands.
- The staff have both the time and the skill to establish a relationship of trust with families.
- The child is seen as a member of the family and the family as part of a community.
- Projects have enthusiastic, committed leadership, clearly specified, measurable aims and focus on families with high levels of need.
- There is a sustained, high quality of input and importantly, sufficient continuity of input to develop a relationship with the individual client.

Screening has been criticized as an unwarranted intrusion into people's lives and a means of extending surveillance over whole populations. The vogue for screening has been interpreted as an example of increased regulation and self-regulation of people within society (Bunton and Burrows, 1995; Lupton, 1995). The scientifically respectable notion of risk assessment justifies more and more investigation and encroachment into people's lifestyles. People are subjected to measurement and the investigation of their lifestyles and behaviours with no immediate benefit to themselves. Whether people have fully consented to the collection of this information is another issue which is debatable.

D   Some firms randomly test their employees for alcohol and illegal drug use. It is a condition of employment that the employee agrees to undertake such tests.
Do you think this policy is:
(a) medically justified?
(b) ethical?

The cost-effectiveness of national screening programmes is much debated. Preventive health services are subject to the inverse-care law, which states that those most in need of the service are least likely to get it (Waller *et al.*, 1990; Griffiths *et al.*, 1994). Planned health promotion activities may reinforce existing inequalities instead of promoting equity (Waller *et al.*, 1990; Gillam, 1992; Griffiths *et al.*, 1994). Costs per case detected through screening may be very high. One estimate is of £300,000 per life saved through cervical screening (Mant and Fowler, 1990). However, once demand has been stimulated by a national campaign, it is difficult to withdraw a screening programme. Screening is generally a popular service, and there is a constant demand for more screening. The costs of a national screening programme are considerable, and have to be offset against other potential uses of the money allocated to screening.

Example

Prostate cancer

Prostate cancer killed 9629 men in 1992, almost all of whom were over 60. Prostate cancer is the second most common form of cancer death in men in the UK and between 1979 and 1988 the number of cases increased by 30%. There is then a considerable argument in favour of finding a reliable method of detection. Arguments against the implementation of a mass screening programme include:

- The expense involved in mass screening.
- There is no effective method of detection. Digital rectal examination is only accurate in 30–40% cases. Blood tests and ultrasound are not very reliable either.
- Because methods of detection are not specific enough to distinguish between benign and malignant tumours, men may have unnecessary surgery, the side-effects of which are severe – 50% becoming impotent, 5% incontinent and 1% may die.

There is very little funding into prostate cancer to identify causes and risk factors or evaluate screening methods or treatment. The main form of prevention then is health education. An HEA campaign is aiming to highlight the risks of prostate cancer and raise awareness of the main symptoms so that men will visit their GP at an early stage when the cancer may be curable.
(Sources: Austoker, 1994; Linehan, 1995.)
How do you account for the lack of action on prostate cancer?

D People of African–Caribbean origin are disproportionately likely to suffer from hypertension. Should the African–Caribbean population be targeted for blood pressure screening? How should this be done – opportunistically, through a call up system, or through referral to a hypertension clinic?

Whole population screening is of debatable value (Goodwin, 1990). In order to justify such a widespread intrusion into people's lives, which has costs of time and money as well as a psychological burden of raised anxiety, the benefits need to outweigh these costs. There is as yet no consensus or definitive evidence to show that wholesale screening is a justifiable policy. Screening more closely targeted populations appears to be a better use of resources. However, there remain many problems of defining at-risk populations and carrying out screening procedures in ways which are acceptable and accessible and which promote health.

PHC and Health for All principles

Health promotion is concerned with the empowerment of individuals and communities to control their own health. But how empowering is the typical experience of attending a PHC surgery or clinic? The setting is dominated by the health professionals whose work base it is. Whilst many surgeries and clinics have tried to become more accessible and friendly, through for example the use of play areas and the provision of health information leaflets and posters, the dominant impression is often that the professionals' work routines take precedence over user preferences. The fact that people attend as individuals makes it difficult for users to share perceptions and make suggestions for change. Statutory services are used to working *for* people, but the experience of working *with* people is novel and requires new skills and changes in how people and organizations work (Taylor, 1996). Participation is typically defined in terms of a participating recipient of services rather than an active participant (Pehl, 1994).

R

> Think back to the last time you attended a PHC surgery or clinic as a patient.
> - What aspects of your visit made you feel more confident and capable of exercising informed choice?
> - What aspects made you feel dependent and vulnerable?
> - Do you think you are a typical user?

Macdonald (1993) argues that PHC in Britain is interpreted in an overly narrow and medical perspective. Health is much more than access to good quality medical services, but for most practitioners, health is subsumed under medicine. By contrast, many developing countries have embraced the WHO's broader idea of PHC which encompasses a social model of health based on the principles of equity, intersectoral collaboration and participation.

Example

Traditional birth attendants

Macdonald (1993) cites the example of traditional birth attendants (TBAs) who are active community partners in healthcare provision. "TBAs are members of the community whose work is esteemed and enhanced through contact with the health services" Macdonald (1993:60). TBAs ensure that birthing experiences benefit from medical knowledge as well as being socially acceptable, and provide a service which is accessible to all women.

Macdonald (1993) argues that these principles are of equal value in developed countries, and should be enshrined in PHC in all countries. This presents a major challenge in Britain where high technology medical expertise dominates the healthcare services. However, the strains upon the system from changing demographics and escalating costs mean that such a re-evaluation is timely. The "Local Voices" NHS initiative, launched in 1992, was intended to give people an effective voice in the shaping of health services locally (NHSME, 1992). The following case study shows how health authorities can facilitate participation and community development to ensure health needs are met in accessible and appropriate ways.

Case study

St Peters, Plymouth

In 1992, a Deprivation Initiative was set up by the Plymouth Health Authority. The target area, St Peters Ward, is an inner-city area highlighted as multiply deprived by data from the Census and the Health Authority. On a variety of indicators, residents had lowered health status. The project's aim was to use a community development approach to involve residents in setting the health agenda and identifying appropriate responses from service providers. The project also aimed to reorientate existing statutory services and make them more reponsive to local needs. An annual budget of £150,000 was allocated and a health visitor appointed as project manager. The project manager undertook a health needs assessment exercise using available data and rapid appraisal methods which involved interviews with key individuals within the community. The project was successful in identifying appropriate action to address identified problems (Table 7.3). Many of these suggestions have now been implemented; some are still in the planning stage.

Table 7.3 *Identified needs and action: St Peters Deprivation Initiative*

Identified need	Action
Need someone to talk to about problems	Plans to change provision of counselling, women's groups
Nowhere to get affordable pregnancy testing and counselling	Free pregnancy testing and counselling at local community development work project
More time with health visitor	Funding to support changes in health visitor working and allow more time
Carers not consulted or involved	Carers impact work in pilot site with long-term aim to involve carers and improve services
Drug and alcohol misuse, particularly amongst young people	Community Development Drug Project with an emphasis on community safety and education, using drama as a tool
Difficult to get to the District General Hospital	Identification of a local site where outpatient and simple diagnostic facilities could be provided
Long wait to see speech therapist, service difficult to access	Reorganization and reorientation of speech and language services. Focus on community-based pro-active role
Need advice about normal and special diets	Community dietitian input to local groups and community-based nutrition project – food co-operative
Antenatal classes stop when baby is born. Services for children with behavioural problems difficult to access, long wait	"Parentwise" project set up to support and empower parents, drawing on community resources. Seeks to be pro-active and to help prevent problems recurring

The project manager reports that five important factors have been highlighted:

- A strong community infrastructure is needed.
- Multi-agency work is vital.
- Flexibility and rapidity of response is crucial.
- Budget allocation probably needs to be increased in stages and ultimately become integrated into mainstream purchasing and contracting of services.
- Evaluation, both qualitative and quantitative, needs to be built into each individual scheme.

Source: Lapthorne, 1996

"The Community Development approach to health is positive and proactive and can enable people to use existing services who do not normally access them. As it seeks to redress the balance and to help communities help themselves, most importantly, it can begin to reduce the inequality and ensure that those with the greatest need have the best care"

(Lapthorne, 1996:39).

Purchasing contracts are driven by clinical effectiveness. The lack of a strong body of evidence on the effectiveness of health promotion in PHC hinders development. The need to determine the effectiveness of health promotion requires a commitment to research in the PHC setting. This is endorsed by the call for evidence-based practice (see Chapter 3). However, embracing Health for All principles in research means challenging the traditional scientific notion of research. These issues are discussed in more detail in Chapter 2.

Adopting the goals of empowerment, participation, equity and intersectoral collaboration would lead to far-reaching changes in the delivery of PHC. This may not be realistic or even desirable. Russell (1995) points out that major changes in practitioners' roles may be inappropriate. There may be a conflict between the values of the individual practitioner/client relationship and those of seeing the practice population's health needs as a whole. Primary healthcare is very good at what it does – treating and managing ill-health. Perhaps it is not appropriate to force changes which jeopardize the central function of PHC.

D

The value of child immunization may differ according to whether the perspective taken is that of the individual patient or the practice population as a whole. Whilst whole population immunization benefits everyone (by reducing the chance of an epidemic), particular individuals may be at risk of developing complications following immunization. Can the two perspectives be reconciled? Which perspective should be paramount in PHC settings?

There are examples of innovative approaches to health promotion in PHC which use Health for All principles (see, for example, the St Peters, Plymouth case study above). Russell (1995) cites examples of community health projects, advice and advocacy projects which focus on the social causes of ill-health, and public health nursing. However, these are the exception rather than the rule. For PHC to embrace Health for All principles would require a massive paradigm shift, or change in the ways of thinking, from a medical individual model of disease to a social collective model of health:

> ". . . our practice area is very hilly and our response to the bronchitic and angina-ridden patients was to increase their medication. The (community health) project's response was to negotiate with the local council to provide a bus route"
>
> (Fisher, cited in Russell, 1995:27).

D How could PHCTs redefine their role to include social advocacy? What problems would this create?

Adopting a social model of health and the principle of participation means taking a lead from local communities and responding to their health concerns. This may take many forms: changing statutory service provision, creating healthy alliances, or supporting and funding community health projects which are independent of the practice.

These fundamental changes can only succeed if supported by an integrated strategic approach (Russell, 1995).

> "A strategy for health promotion in primary care ... is more than the aggregate of individual activities within the practice. It implies a targeted, multifaceted approach to the practice population based on a shared practice view of priorities for improving the health of that population"
>
> (Doyle and Thomas, 1996:7).

Strategy implies

- shared guiding principles;
- continuity;
- integration.

We have already stated that Health for All principles provide appropriate guidelines to inform practice. However, these principles do not guide the present allocation of resources for health promotion in PHC. In particular, channelling resources and accountability through GPs is not appropriate, given their primary role. Health visitors or public health nurses, with their training in population health, may be more appropriate lead practitioners for health promotion (Russell, 1995; Doyle and Thomas, 1996; Orme and Wright, 1996).

Continuity depends on adequate funding. Innovative health promotion projects are unlikely to be securely supported through long-term ring-fenced funding. Specialist health promotion services which co-ordinate and advise on PHC interventions provide a valuable resource, but one which may not be considered a priority or be purchased by commissioning authorities. A major barrier to integration is the mismatch of resources and collaboration between primary care and public health (Doyle and Thomas, 1996). Funding for public health and health promotion is a fraction of that for medical treatment. Resourcing health in PHC requires a more widespread and flexible funding system which supports not only PHC practitioners but also specialist health promotion services and community health projects.

At the level of PHC, integration relies on teamwork, healthy alliances and shared training and research. These issues are discussed in more detail in Chapter 8. PHC networks have sprung up throughout the country and provide a forum for integration of activities (HEA, 1995).

Even if all the above principles were to be adopted by PHCTs, delivering health promotion through PHC can never be the whole answer. The small minority of people not registered with GPs includes those with significant health needs, for example, homeless people and travellers, refugees and people with mental illness (Russell, 1995). Conventional PHC health promotion needs a safety net of community provision in order to reach the whole population.

Conclusion

There are many sound reasons for promoting health in PHC settings. However there are also many practical problems with ensuring health promotion is prioritized within PHC. These result from the pressures facing PHC practitioners and their primary role to treat and prevent ill-health. There are, in addition, fundamental problems deriving from the particular perspective of PHC practitioners which favours individual-based medical care over population-based public healthcare. Embracing the core principles of the WHO's Health for All programme within PHC is difficult, given its traditional focus on expert medical diagnosis and treatment of individual patients.

Two approaches to health promotion in PHC have been outlined in this chapter. One calls for a major reconstruction of PHC services to bring them more into line with HFA principles (Macdonald, 1993). The other proposes that PHC and GPs should not be the central focus for health promotion resourcing (Russell, 1995). Given the unlikelihood of major changes in training, structure or perspective of the PHC services in Britain, the PHC setting has inevitable limitations. There are, however, certain advantages in promoting health through PHC services, and it appears that such activities can be effective in reducing mortality and morbidity and in promoting quality of life. It would therefore seem to be a worthwhile enterprise to maximize the health promotion potential of PHC services. This requires, as a minimum, a co-ordinated and resourced strategy which seeks to go beyond the medical model of health.

Further discussion

■ What features of PHC in Britain support the principles of empowerment, equity, intersectoral collaboration and participation?
■ Can you think of any examples?
■ What features of PHC present barriers to these principles?

Recommended reading

■ Macdonald J J (1993) *Primary health care: Medicine in its place*, London, Earthscan.
  A detailed discussion of the need to adopt the WHO's broader definition of PHC which is based on HFA principles. A global perspective is used.

■ Russell J (1995) *A review of health promotion in primary care*, London, The Greater London Association of Community Health Councils.
  A critical review which questions whether the 1993 GP banding arrangements for health promotion in PHC are the best use of resources.

References

Atkin K and Hirst M (1994) *Costing practice nurses: Implications for primary health* care, Discussion Paper 17, York, Centre of Health Economics, University of York.

Austoker H (1994) "Screening for ovarian, prostatic and testicular cancer", *British Medical Journal*, **309**, 315–320.

Bunton R and Burrows R (1995) "Consumption and health in the 'epidemiological' clinic of late modern medicine", in Bunton R, Nettleton S and Burrows R (eds), *The sociology of health promotion: Critical analyses of consumption, lifestyle and risk*, pp. 206–22, London, Routledge.

Commission on Chronic Illness (1957) *Chronic illness in the United States: Vol. I Prevention of chronic illness*, Cambridge, Mass., Harvard University Press.

Coronary Prevention Group (1993) *Nutrition interventions in primary health care: A literature review*, London, Health Education Authority Briefing Paper.

Cupples ME, McKnight A, O'Neill C and Normand C (1996) "The effect of personal health education on the quality of life of patients with angina in general practice", *Health Education Journal*, **55**(1), 75–83.

Daykin N, Naidoo J and Wilson N (1995) *Effective health promotion in primary health care: A resource for primary health care workers*, Bristol, Faculty of Health and Social Care, University of the West of England.

Daykin N and Naidoo J (1997) "Poverty and health promotion in primary health care: Professional perspectives", *Health and Social Care in the Community*, **5**, 309–317.

Doxiadis S (1987) *Ethical dilemmas in health promotion*, London, Wiley.

Doyle Y and Thomas P (1996) "Promoting health

through primary care: challenges in taking a strategic approach", *Health Education Journal*, **55**, 3–10.

Editorial (1996) "New health promotion deal for GPs", *Healthlines*, July/August, 4.

Family Heart Study Group (1994) "Randomised control trial evaluating cardiovascular screening and intervention in general practice: principal results of British family heart study", *British Medical Journal*, **308**, 313-20.

Gillam S (1992) "The provision of health promotion clinics in relation to population need: another example of the inverse care law?", *British Journal of General Practice*, **42**, 54–56.

Goodwin S (1990) "Setting the scene: is screening health promotion?", in Thompson J and Brown B *Screening and Health Promotion Seminar*, pp. 9–16, Blackpool, Wyre and Fylde Health Authority.

Gregson BA, Cartlidge AM and Bond J (1992) "Development of a measure of professional collaboration in primary health care", *Journal of Epidemiology and Community Health*, **46**, 48–53.

Griffiths C, Cooke S and Toon P (1994) "Registration health checks: inverse care in the inner city?", *British Journal of General Practice*, **44**, 201–4.

Hall DMB (ed.) (1996) *Health for all children: Report of the third joint working party on child health surveillance*, 3rd edn, Oxford, Oxford University Press.

Hasler JC (1994) *The primary health care team*, London, John Fry Trust Fellowship/Royal Society of Medicine Press.

Health Education Authority (1995) *Health promotion in primary health care: the way forward: Report on two one-day networking events for purchasers and providers of health promotion in primary care*, London, Health Education Authority.

Kaufman A (1990) "GPs crack under constant stress", *Physician* **9**, 632–35.

Lapthorne D (1996) "St Peters, Plymouth", in Burton P and Harrison L (eds) *Identifying local health needs: New community based approaches*, Bristol, The Policy Press.

Larner M *et al.* (1992) *Fair start for children – lessons learnt from seven demonstration projects*, Connecticut, Yale University Press.

Linehan T (1995) "Preventing prostate cancer: to screen or not to screen", *Healthlines*, October, 17–19.

Lupton D (1995) *The imperative of health: public health and the regulated body*, London, Sage.

Macdonald JJ (1993) *Primary health care: Medicine in its place*, London, Earthscan.

MacPherson K (1994) "The evidence for a population approach to uni and multifactorial interventions in primary care – Where do OXCHECK and FHS fit", in *Cardiovascular prevention in primary care: The way forwards*, London, Kings Fund.

Mant and Fowler (1990) *British Medical Journal*, **300**, 916–18.

NHS Executive (1995) *Developing NHS purchasing and GP fundholding: Towards a primary care-led NHS*, Leeds, NHS.

NHSME (1992) *Local voices: the views of local people in purchasing for health*, London, Department of Health.

Office of Health Economics (1994) *Health information and the consumer*, OHE Briefing no. 30, York, Office of Health Economics.

Orme J and Wright C (1996) "Health promotion in primary health care", in Scriven A and Orme J (eds) *Health promotion: Professional perspectives*, pp. 54–65, Basingstoke, Macmillan Press and Open University.

OXCHECK Study Group (1994) "Effectiveness of health checks conducted by nurses in primary care: results of the OXCHECK study after one year", *British Medical Journal*, **308**, 308–12.

OXCHECK Study Group (1995) "The effectiveness of health checks conducted by nurses in primary care: final results from the OXCHECK study", *British Medical Journal*, **310**, 1099–104.

Pehl L (1994) *The development of effective evaluation for health promotion activity within the new GP contract*, South Thames Regional Health Authority.

Prochaska JO and DiClemente C (1984) *The transtheoretical approach: Crossing traditional foundations of change*, Homewood, Illinois, Don Jones/Irwin.

Royal College of General Practitioners and Office of Population Censuses and Surveys (1986) *Morbidity Statistics from General Practice 1981–2: Third National Survey*, DHSS series MB5, No. 1, London, HMSO.

Russel M, Wilson C, Taylor C, Baker C (1979)

"Effectiveness of general practitioners' advice against smoking", *British Medical Journal*, **2**, 231–35.

Russell J (1995) *A review of health promotion in primary care*, London, The Greater London Association of Community Health Councils.

Taylor D and Bloor K (1994) *Health care, health promotion and the future general practice*, London, The Nuffield Provincial Hospitals Trust/Royal Society of Medicine Press.

Taylor P (1996) "Supporting community involvement: the organisational challenges", in Burton P and Harrison L (eds) *Identifying local health needs: New community based approaches*, Bristol, The Policy Press.

Waller D *et al.* (1990) "Health checks in general practice: another example of inverse care?", *British Medical Journal*, **300**, 1115–18.

Williams S, Calnan M, Cant L and Coyle J (1993) "All change in the NHS?: Implications of the NHS reforms for primary care prevention," *Sociology of Health and Illness*, **15**, 43–67.

Wilson A, McDonald P, Hayes L and Cooney J (1992) "Health promotion in the general practice consultation: a minute makes a difference", *British Medical Journal*, **304**, 227–30.

Wilson Barnett J and Macleod Clark J (eds) (1993) *Research in health promotion nursing*, London, Macmillan.

Wonderling D, Langham S, Buxton M, Normand C and McDermott C (1996) "What can be concluded from the Oxcheck and British family heart studies: commentary on cost effectiveness analyses", *British Medical Journal*, **312**, 1274–78.

WHO (1978) *Report on the primary health care conference: Alma Ata*, Geneva, WHO.

Yen L (1995) "From Alma Ata to Asda – and beyond: a commentary on the transition in health promotion services in primary care from commodity to control", in Bunton R, Nettleton S and Burrows R (eds) *The sociology of health promotion: Critical analyses of consumption, lifestyle and risk*, London, Routledge.

8 *Collaboration for health promotion*

Key points

- Defining intersectoral collaboration.
- The impetus for collaboration:
  - National health strategy;
  - Healthy public policy.
- Theoretical frameworks for intersectoral collaboration:
  - organizational theory;
  - groupwork theory.

Overview

Building a supportive physical, cultural and socio-economic environment for people to live and work is deemed one of the most important purposes of health promotion according to the Ottawa Charter (WHO, 1986). It is based on the understanding that individual and community well-being is determined more by social, environmental and economic systems than healthcare provision. It follows then that the promotion and maintenance of health does not belong to one professional group or sector. The WHO state that intersectoral collaboration across different public sectors is central to achieving the goal of Health For All and to the development of a healthy public policy.

The "Health of the Nation" strategy for England in 1992 reinforced the importance of practitioners working together, and the revised strategy "Our Healthier Nation" also supports the concept of broad healthy alliances as the key way to deliver health improvement. This chapter looks at the context in which the current emphasis on collaboration has arisen and explores the tensions underpinning current practice. It outlines how an understanding of organizational theory and groupwork theory can help to identify key themes in successful collaborative working.

Introduction

The Department of Health has used the term "healthy alliance" to define the way agencies can work together to promote health, emphazising co-operation and partnership:

> "A healthy alliance is in effect a partnership of individuals and organizations formed to enable people to increase their influence over the factors that affect their health and well being"
> (DoH, 1993:22).

In "Working Together for Better Health", published in 1993, the Department of Health suggest that the advantages of collaborative activity include:

- a wider pool of knowledge and experience;
- more effective use of resources;
- increased access to networks;
- more significant achievements through joint working than by agencies working separately.

A further example of the degree of commitment by the Department of Health to this way of working and an incentive to organizations is the establishment of national and regional awards for healthy alliances based on good practice and for which there are limited cash prizes (see p. 166).

The WHO used the term "Intersectoral Collaboration" to emphasize that collaboration should take place across public sectors and involve a wide range of agencies. The Alma Ata declaration (WHO, 1978) stated that health could only be attained by action in spheres additional to the health sector, in particular: agriculture, animal husbandry, food industry, education, housing, public works and communications. The Healthy Cities initiative set up in 1987 to work towards Health For All aimed to establish healthy public policies in cities, co-ordinating services and policy decisions. In 1990 a survey of District and Regional Health Authorities found that 80% claimed to have established partnerships with other agencies to work towards Health For All (Institute of Health Service Managers, 1990). Local Authorities were cited as the most frequent partners followed by voluntary organizations. A survey by the Health Education Authority in 1992 found 140 cases of collaboration between NHS sectors and voluntary organizations (Fieldgrass, 1992). Collaboration between organizations in order to promote health thus has a high profile. In this chapter we shall discuss what might lie behind this public commitment to inter-agency working.

Although intersectoral collaboration is a key principle of Health For All and endorsed in the national health strategy, to expect it to happen automatically is unrealistic. Indeed many practitioners' experience of collaborative working is of intense competition and rivalry and a reluctance to share information or "give up" areas of work. Added to this are the differing perspectives that organizations have on what exactly constitutes promoting health. There is no identifiable theory of collaboration which can help to illuminate this.

"Collaboration is a paradoxical concept in the field of social welfare. There can be little doubt that the notion is in vogue. The desirability of some form of collaborative activity has become a *sine qua non* of effective practice within the welfare professions, both at practitioner and policy making levels. However we know remarkably little about how collaborative activity works, why it may initially be developed, how it may be measured or even how it may be defined"

(Hudson, 1987:145).

There are only a small number of studies which focus on collaborative activity and these are principally in the fields of child protection where inter-agency co-operation is a high priority (Department of Health, 1991; Birchall and Hallett, 1992) and the working of primary healthcare teams (Ovreteit, 1993). There are a few empirical studies in the UK of intersectoral collaboration in the health promotion field which attempt to develop a theory of collaboration (Davies *et al.*, 1993; Delaney, 1994a; Springett, 1995) but otherwise most of the conclusions about the features of successful collaboration draw mainly on the experience of practitioners. This chapter draws on organizational studies and groupwork theory to explore why collaboration is a difficult principle to put into practice.

Defining intersectoral collaboration

The fact that the WHO use the term "collaboration" and the Department of Health use the term "healthy alliance" illustrates the terminological confusion that exists in describing health and welfare practitioners working together. Table 8.1 shows the distinctions made by Leathard (1994) between

- concept-based terms;
- process-based terms;
- agency-based terms.

Concept-based terms include those most commonly used in the health sector of "interdisciplinary" or "multidisciplinary" working. These terms both refer to a team of individuals with different professional or training backgrounds (e.g. nursing, education, social work) who make different contributions to the team. Interdisciplinary means within the same professional group, e.g. community nurses and acute sector nurses, whereas multidisciplinary is normally taken to refer to a wider group which includes members from different professions.

As can be seen from the terms used to describe the ways agencies work together, intersectoral collaboration can take place at many levels:

- The day-to-day liaison that takes place between health and social care professionals about clients and service delivery with the intention of seamless care.

Table 8.1 *Alternative terms used variously for inter-professional work denoting learning together and working together*

Concept-based	Process-based	Agency-based
Interdisciplinary	Joint planning	Inter-agency
Multidisciplinary	Joint training	Intersectoral
Multiprofessional	Shared learning	Trans-sectoral
Transprofessional	Teamwork	Cross-agency
Transdisciplinary	Partnership	Consortium
Holistic	Merger	Commission
Generic	Groupwork	Healthy alliances
	Collaboration	Forum
	Integration	Alliance
	Co-operation	Centre
	Liaison	Federation
	Synergy	Confederation
	Bonding	Inter-institutional
	Common core	Locality groups
	Interlinked	
	Interrelated	
	Joint project	
	Collaborative care planning	
	Locality planning	
	Unification	
	Co-ordination	
	Multilateral	
	Joint learning	
	Joint management	
	Joint budgets	
	Working interface	
	Participation	
	Collaborative working	
	Involvement	
	Joint working	
	Jointness	

Reproduced from Leathard (1994), with permission

- The formal arrangements that exist for the planning of service delivery such as Joint Care Planning.
- Formal arrangements to co-ordinate the collection of information such as a Substance Misuse Reference Group or the data linkage project described in Chapter 9.
- Inter-agency working groups on issues of shared concern or collaborative projects.
- The co-ordination of policy and priorities across key agencies such as Healthy Cities initiatives or the transport initiatives described in Chapter 10.

Alliances can be:

- loose networks or formal arrangements;

- single issue or broad based;
- have a fixed timescale or an ongoing remit;
- neighbourhood, community or nationally based and be concerned with a client group, a health issue or broader issues such as environmental responsibility.

The partners in an alliance are determined largely by the nature of the task and how broadly the co-ordinating agency interprets "health". Likely partners for alliances include the Health Education Authority, Local Authorities, voluntary organizations, and the media and settings which contribute to health such as schools, cities and workplaces.

In Table 8.1 there are many process based terms to describe working together. Many of these terms are used synonymously although there are differences. Ovreteit (1993) when discussing how people from different professions and agencies work together gives emphasis to three key words:

- Co-ordinate – to bring into order as parts of a whole.
- Collaborate – to labour together, to act jointly.
- Co-operate – to unite for a common effort and shared goals.

Co-operative and collaborative working thus need to be distinguished from co-ordination, which is the term used to describe "corporate approaches" in which there is a mandated authority to co-operate. For example, the latter applies in Community Care Plans between Health Authorities and Social Services (Davies *et al.*, 1993) where there needs to be clear goals and structures for co-ordination. Ovreteit also distinguishes between collaboration, in which partners work together but do not necessarily agree, and co-operation in which joint working is for a common goal.

Table 8.2 cites some examples of public sector collaboration. It shows how the main impetus for collaboration between Health Authorities and Local Authorities has been to provide planned and "seamless" services in health and social welfare. The need for urban regeneration has provided the impetus and various cash incentives (e.g. Single Regeneration Budgets) for businesses, voluntary and community groups and Local Authorities to work together to develop social and planning policies which address housing, transport,crime and opportunities for social networks.

National health strategy

The "Health of the Nation" strategy document adopted the term "healthy alliance" to denote partnerships to promote health. The Department of Health can point to numerous examples of healthy

> **R** Think of an "alliance" in which you are a partner. How would you describe its main purpose?

Table 8.2 *The impetus to intersectoral and inter-agency collaboration*

(1) A shift in emphasis from the acute sector to the community health sector with an emphasis on primary healthcare teams, e.g.:
1981   "Care in Action" "Care in the Community"
1986   Cumberlege report
1986   Project 2000 nurse training establishing common paths in community nursing
(2) Public inquiries into child abuse cases (Beckford, 1985; Kimberley Carlisle, 1987; Cleveland, 1987) which highlighted a lack of co-ordination between relevant agencies – doctors, health visitors, social workers, the police, courts, school welfare and teachers, e.g.:
1989   Children Act
1991   Department of Health policy guidelines "Working Together: a guide to Arrangements for Inter-Agency Cooperation for the Protection of Children from Abuse"
(3) The need for better cooperation between health and social services to provide care in the community, particularly for the elderly, disabled and mentally ill, e.g.:
1990   NHS and Community Care Act
This legislation has also influenced joint hospital discharge policies, joint purchasing between health authorities, mergers between social service departments and housing and sometimes between social services and education and between health authorities and Family Health Service Authorities.

alliances. There were, for example, 300 alliances representing over 2000 organizations which entered the 1996 healthy alliance awards offered by the Department of Health. The winners included:

- "Heartwell", a scheme to encourage heart health activities in organizations in South Humberside;
- a cancer awareness teaching pack for schools in the London Borough of Barnet;
- a Redbridge home safety campaign which brought in Eastern Electricity plc to install safety products and Help The Aged to offer home safety advice to older people;
- the "Stepping Stones" project in Lancashire in which Social and Health services and voluntary groups help people with mental health problems return to education.

These examples show how the NHS has many potential partners in promoting health. Historically, health was part of Local Authority activity but since the inception of the NHS in 1948 many of those public health functions have been taken over. However, local authorities retain many functions which clearly impact on the health of the population:

- housing;
- education;
- environment including planning, road safety, traffic management, air quality (although road planning is the responsibility of the Department of Transport);
- leisure facilities and adult education;
- consumer protection including food hygiene;
- health and safety at work.

The endorsement of intersectoral collaboration within the "Health of the Nation" could have provided the opportunity for a broad approach to health promotion with common goals across all public sectors; instead the "Health of the Nation" endorsed the concept of "partnership". Whilst in some cases this moved joint working from the operational and practitioner level to the strategic level, in many cases "healthy alliances" did not lead to new sorts of work. They have merely formalized the partnerships which previously existed such as the links between health promotion departments and schools. Studies of alliances have shown that in many instances their development has been incremental and informal – with one working partnership leading to more general collaboration (Springett, 1995). Much of what goes under the name of a healthy alliance is not at all "healthy" in achieving collaboration and is merely a co-ordinating mechanism to exchange information. The new Labour government has a broader approach. For the first time, there is a minister in the Department of Health whose responsibility is exclusively public health. But health is also seen as the function of every other government department.

Despite the vital role of Local Authorities in promoting health, the relationship beween Health Authorities and councils has not been easy. In the past, the work has been dominated by Health Authorities, and the Local Authorities have been the unequal partners in healthy alliances.

D

"The general pattern of collaboration would seem to be one of the health service eliciting support of other sectors for the implementation of NHS initiated policies"

(Farrant, 1986).

Do you agree with the above statement? Can you identify any changes in collaborative working since 1986?

One of the main changes in collaborative working is that Health Authorities and Local Authorities are involved in ensuring that services are available rather than necessarily providing them. So collaboration becomes a necessity for patients discharged into the community but is still not evident over broader public health concerns.

Financial resources used to act as an incentive for Health Authorities and Local Authorities to collaborate. Joint financing was started in 1976 to offer short-term support for specific projects selected by both sectors which would then be funded by the Local Authority. In practice, as Hogg (1991:65) points out "it often appeared as if the Health Authority was trying to transfer responsibility to the Local Authority". There is no specific funding for alliances set up under the "Health of the Nation" and the use of one-off grants (e.g. Home Office Drug Prevention Initiative, Safe Cities, City Challenge) can lead to competition between projects which share the same broad aims, e.g. reducing inequalities.

The NHS reforms have had a huge impact on organizational arrangements and therefore on the ways in which sectors can work together. Ewles cites a number of challenges to the rhetoric of healthy alliances (Ewles, 1993, 1996).

- Competition between provider health authorities bidding against each other to provide services.
- The need for both purchasers and provider health authorities to be part of many alliances. Some of these may already be in a contractual arrangement adding an "uncomfortable dynamic" to an alliance.
- The selling off of core services of Local Authorities such as leisure services and school catering, making co-ordinated health promotion more difficult.
- The lack of co-terminosity between Local Authorities and Health Authorities requiring, in many cases, at least two Trusts or two Local Authorities to be present in alliances. The boundaries also being too large to allow for links with the community.

Under the framework of the "Health of the Nation" strategy, the alliances that were formed were primarily to develop strategies for healthier lifestyles and did not address structural concerns. The understanding of collaboration focused on NHS control, articulating a medical model of health (Davies *et al.*, 1993). The new Labour government has reiterated the importance of local collaboration and for government departments to liaise together to ensure that all policies take account of their impact on health.

"On the one hand, the Health of the Nation presents opportunities for interagency working – acknowledging that health is determined by factors beyond the control or responsibility of the NHS and providing Health Authorities with an explicit directive to establish healthy alliances. However, on the other hand, it also presents a potential threat to existing collaborative working: articulating a medical model of health; an NHS dominated agenda with targets focused primarily on disease, prevention and individual lifestyles; and an understanding of collaboration focused on NHS control"

(Davies *et al.*, 1993).

Healthy public policy

There is considerable evidence that low income, inadequate diet, poor housing , environmental pollution and lack of access to health-care are factors which contribute to persistent health inequalities and deprivation (e.g. Benzeval, Judge and Whitehead, 1995). This awareness of the factors contributing to the nation's health has been characterized as the "new public health movement". What is new about this movement is the "(re-) discovery that threats to the population's health are heterogeneous and multi-dimensional" (Scambler and Goraya, 1994). It is a rediscovery in the sense that promoting health through public policy is not new. The nineteenth century saw the development of the "sanitary idea", a recognition that over-crowding in insanitary conditions was the cause of major epidemics and illness in the Victorian towns. By the 1920s breakthroughs in pharmacology (e.g. insulin, penicillin) gave rise to the dominance of medicine. A reappraisal of the scope for improved health through changing environments only emerged again in the 1970s (Ashton and Seymour, 1988). The threats to the nation's health are multi-dimensional in the sense that many of the issues which are of most current concern involve agencies and sectors beyond the NHS. The Black Report, for example, which highlighted the links between deprivation and health chose the abolition of child poverty as the most important national goal for health (Townsend and Davidson, 1982).

Whereas the nineteenth century public health movement focused on disease prevention through environmental measures, the new public health movement aims to intervene in all areas of public policy which influence health. The 1988 World Health Organization conference in Adelaide on healthy public policy saw the need for health awareness to be "threaded through" all government departments.

> "Healthy public policy is the policy challenge set by a new vision of public health. It refers to policy decisions in any sector or level of government that are characterized by an explicit concern for health and an accountability for health impact. It is expressed through horizontal strategies such as intersectoral collaboration and public participation"

(WHO, 1988).

D The Labour government has stated that policies concerning the economy, income support, transport, housing, agriculture and the environment are to be perceived as health issues. How do you account for the separation there has been of health issues from public policy?

Agenda 21

An agreement on the need for sustaining the environment was reached at the Earth Summit in Rio de Janeiro in 1992. Under the 1993 UK strategy for Sustainable Development, Local Authorities are required to publish Agenda 21 strategies on how to protect the environment for the twenty first century. The growing consumption of resources, particularly by the developed countries of the north, pose substantial risks to the environment and to public health through the depletion of finite resources, increased pollution of air, land and water and increased waste. Agenda 21 commits governments to the following objectives on health:

- Meeting the basic prerequisites for health, e.g. access to safe food and water, sanitation and housing.
- Controlling communicable diseases.
- Protecting vulnerable groups such as children and older people.
- Reducing the health risks caused by pollution, excessive energy consumption and waste.

This is a global action plan but it recognizes that protecting the environment starts in local communities improving their neighbourhood and planning for the future. The Public Health Alliance describes a sustainable community as one which accepts "stewardship of its surroundings and uses its own resources, both physical and social, to meet its own needs" (Crombie, 1996). The link between these concerns about the environment and public health was made closer by the incorporation into the "Health of the Nation" of a sixth key area on the environment. Initially, this was to focus on:

- outdoor air quality (including lead, sulfur dioxide and ozone emissions);
- indoor air quality (including cigarette smoke and nitrogen dioxide from gas cookers);
- radon (a natural radioactive gas linked to lung cancer);
- noise;
- lead in drinking water.

The new Labour government is to extend this remit to cover the impact on health from poor housing, transport and food safety.

Working towards sustainable development thus demands collaboration across public, private and voluntary sectors and the involvement of agencies which may not see themselves as primarily health oriented. In Luton, for example, Local Authority environmental services and the planning department have led borough-wide consultations with business and community groups and the Health Authority on what life would be like in Luton in the twenty first century. Five priorities emerged: economic prosperity and work opportunities, quality of life, the town's environment and its energy use, pollution control and waste management, transport and community participation. Agenda 21 thus provides new opportunities for Local Authorities and Health Authorities to work together and for local people to become involved in planning for their community. The focus of activity may be as it was in the nineteenth century around environmental hazards, but it may also encompass, as in Luton's priorities, action to address social influences on health such as employment and income and attempts to create social support networks in the community.

The structural and contextual factors of national policy initiatives and the general economic climate are thus important in contributing to intersectoral collaboration. Health promoters seeking to create and sustain collaboration face a challenging task. The next section reviews two theoretical frameworks which illuminate the processes involved in intersectoral collaboration – organizational theory and groupwork theory.

Theoretical frameworks for intersectoral collaboration

Applying organizational theory

Although little is known about collaboration for health promotion, there is a substantive body of theory on inter-organizational co-ordination in general which suggests that organizations have conflicting interests and degrees of power. Another body of literature on occupational cultures suggests that professions are basically autonomous and resistant to crossing boundaries. The assumption then that organizations can, and want, to work together is somewhat unrealistic. The concept of exchange is therefore seen as the key to understanding collaboration. Regardless of the overt purpose of an organization (e.g. to provide services or meet client needs), most organizations are also concerned to preserve their interests – to ensure adequate resources, their autonomy, status and authority. Working with other agencies results in some loss of independence and control and necessitates the investment of scarce resources into building partnerships, the outcomes of which are by no means clear. Consequently, organizations only enter into collaborative working if they can see the needs of their organization are being met and will benefit in some way.

The Department of Health (1993) identified the following benefits from collaborative working:

- sharing and exchange of information;
- synergy – the effect of collaboration being greater than the work of individual agencies alone;
- effective use of resources through sharing the load; avoiding duplication;
- a range of perspectives and mutual education about ways of working and awareness of issues;

- consistency of message;
- more appropriate targeting and increased access to target groups;
- enhanced credibility;
- putting health on the agenda of organizations which might not see this as their role.

R How does or might your organization benefit from inter-agency working? Are there any of the benefits identified above?

One of the key factors in effective collaboration is achieving an inter-agency equilibrium when power is balanced among the participating agencies. The source of power for an organization varies. Local authorities are controlled by elected politicians; voluntary organizations are accountable to management committees and their client group, health authorities have no direct local accountability. The different basis of Local Authority and Health Authority membership can create different priorities. Local Authority officers who have to work from election to election can find longer-term strategic planning difficult (Delaney, 1994b). Health Authorities are appointed bodies whose accountability for services is governed by the Patient's Charter and various statutory responsibilities but which have only recently embraced the principle of participation and the need for consultation.

D   What factors might constitute "power" for an organization in an alliance?

Power might include information, access to important networks or groups the organization is intended to serve and, crucially, sources of funding. Power also manifests itself in alliances through the way participating organizations negotiate the remit of the alliance and whether they are "invited" to join an alliance by a lead agency. This can lead to the work and contribution of partners not being equally valued.

C ase study

Ageing Well

Consider this case study of Ageing Well, a national healthy alliance involving public, private and voluntary sectors. Do you think Ageing Well could achieve inter-agency equilibrium?

Ageing Well is supported by funds from the Department of Health and two corporate sponsors, a pharmaceutical company and a medical insurance company. It is co-ordinated by a voluntary agency, Age Concern and also receives the contacts, training, research and campaign resources of the Health Education Authority. Its aim is to promote good working relationships between agencies and individuals who work to improve and maintain the health of older people and to encourage older people themselves to become involved in encouraging positive health among their peers by recruiting and training senior health mentors (source: Ashton, 1995).

The exchange theory of organizational relations suggests that for partnerships to develop there needs to be some brokerage and matchmaking, recognizing what each brings to the task and negotiating on points of conflict. Voluntary sector organizations sometimes find it difficult to be active partners in alliances. They are unable to commit any funds to joint working and their organizational culture is different from the statutory and private sectors. Although they are not bound by the roles of the statutory sector, they may be perceived as amateurish and as not accountable. Representatives from the statutory sector, by contrast, have access to core funding and a huge network of contacts which Springett (1995) regards as an important element in alliances and their influence. Many Healthy Cities projects have, however, chosen to site themselves within voluntary organizations because they are perceived as relatively free from bureaucratic structures and power conflicts. The role of voluntary organizations in enabling community involvement is also valued in alliances.

A greater understanding of how other organizations work is often cited as a benefit of collaboration and conversely, a lack of appreciation of others' organizational domains and tasks is cited as a barrier (Davies *et al.*, 1993). Powell (1992) found that to be effective, partners in an alliance need to discover how each others' organizations are structured; how decisions are taken and by whom; their financial and planning processes and the ways in which information is communicated. This vital stage may be overlooked when alliances see their priority as getting things done.

Example

Organizational cultures

A recognition of different organizational cultures is an important element in the understanding of the partners in an alliance. Handy (1976) has identified organizations like tribes and families with their own ways of doing things. He uses the symbolism of four gods to describe the varying types of management that can be discerned in organizations:

- **The club culture symbolized by Zeus.** This organization is characteristic of small family type companies. Control is exercised from the centre with little bureaucracy.
- **The role culture symbolized by Apollo.** This a typical bureaucracy with different departments for different functions such as finance, purchasing, marketing, etc. These are co-ordinated by a hierarchy of managers.
- **The task culture symbolized by Athena.** This is a matrix organization with a team culture. Expertise rather than position is important and management is flat and low key.
- **The existential culture symbolized by Dionysus.** This organization is a cluster of individuals, each of whom is fairly autonomous.

To which culture does your organization belong? How does the leadership and decision making in this kind of culture affect partnerships with other organizations?

The fragmentation and compartmentalizing of practitioners and services which is typical of the role culture of the NHS can make collaboration difficult. Those working in the NHS may be particularly bound by their roles and hierarchical structures. Participants may lack the status to make decisions or commit money or be unclear about the roles of other departments within the organization. Alliance representatives who are committed to the partnership and who share the same values as the other members may not be representative of their organization. Glover describes a workplace project in which "building on an individual's enthusiasm without getting the agreement of the organization they represented created a problem. Consequently, when there were changes of personnel, commitment to the project was lost and support had to be renegotiated with the individual's successor" (Glover, 1996:213). Where alliances have a strategic role, partners need to have enough influence within their own organization to secure a commitment to the policy.

Ensuring that members are representative of the groups to which they belong is particularly difficult when community involvement is emphasized. Community participation is easy to espouse and hard to achieve. In many alliances, participation means merely consultation. Where there is involvement it may be that of "established voices" (e.g. user groups, residents' associations, voluntary agencies) or personal contacts of the professional members of the alliance which serve only to reinforce the marginal nature of disadvantaged groups.

For participants to believe that the alliance is beneficial, there needs to be a clear vision of what it is intended to achieve (Powell, 1992; DoH, 1993; Delaney, 1994a; Nutbeam, 1994). As we saw in Chapter 1, there is no single explanation or definition of what health promotion is, nor any agreed set of principles. When alliances to promote health try to identify their goals, this lack of agreement comes to the fore with competing rationales. Delaney thus calls the basis for developing a shared vision in many alliances "rather flimsy" (Delaney, 1994a:220). Taking the time to identify shared values and a common starting point through workshops and open discussions is deemed to be the first task of an alliance (Powell, 1992).

Activity

In 1985 the Advisory Council on the Misuse of Drugs advised the setting up of District Drug Advisory Committees, an attempt to involve many agencies in drug prevention and treatment. Most DDACs were dominated by Health Authorities and became ineffective talking shops. The government strategy "Tackling Drugs Together 1995–1998" laid down that there should be a new initiative with the emphasis on education and prevention to reduce the acceptability and availability of drugs especially for young people. Agencies should be brought together in Drug Action Teams.

- What agencies might be expected to be part of Drug Action Teams?
- In what ways might these agencies differ in their perspectives on drug prevention?
- How might the agencies' role and remit affect how they view the tasks of the Drug Action Teams?
- How can health promotion objectives be prioritized over safety concerns?
- Given the high profile of drugs issues, how could the Drug Action Teams ensure that they achieve an inter-agency equilibrium?

Participants have to relinquish some control in joint working. For professions in health and welfare which have been seeking to define their professional competence and difference such as nurses and Health Promotion Specialists, crossing professional boundaries and finding ways to work together can be challenging. Beattie (1994) cites the following as common barriers to intersectoral working: (i) professional ambition and competition; (ii) territoriality and protectionism; (iii) information used as a major source of power and shared only reluctantly; (iv) different terminology and jargon. The experience of primary healthcare teams has also shown how relative status and pay can act as a barrier to joint working (West and Slater, 1996).

Reciprocity or mutual exchange is central to intersectoral collaboration. Yet this is the inherent contradiction in the enthusiasm for healthy alliances in the NHS. Whilst networking and collaboration is very much part of the way health promoters work, the NHS reforms have encouraged a different ethos. The establishment of the market and the purchase of services means it is competition not collaboration which underpins the NHS. Equally, the rational planning entailed in healthy alliances may conflict with the informal networks which may have arisen between sectors (Scriven, 1995; Bloxham, 1996).

Using groupwork theory

Most studies on inter-agency working have concentrated on the structures of organizations and the context in which it takes place. Nevertheless most partners in alliances attribute their success or failure to "personalities" and individual members. Whilst the role of personalities can be overplayed, most studies suggest that "networking" is at the heart of collaboration and that nurturing relationships is crucial. Group theory can help us to understand how networking takes place, how groups can fail to achieve their task, and how conflict can arise.

D What reasons might there be for conflict in joint working?

As we saw in the previous section, organizations have partisan interests and want to hold on to their resources and autonomy. In addition, there are professional constraints on collaboration. Health and welfare professions are not given to positive mutual awareness and there is often an assumption that one group may be empire-building or lack commitment. Lack of role clarity is often cited as an explanation for conflict when members aren't clear about their contribution or that of others. Sentiments such as these are commonplace:

- "I don't know what I'm doing here or why I've been invited. I've got nothing to do with health."
- "The Health Authority (or any of the other participants) are just doing this to get more money for themselves."
- "This is just a talking shop. It's got nothing to do with our priorities."

Simnett (1995:156) states:

"Once members of a team understand how they can best contribute to a team, in terms of their roles and know they are valued for their unique contributions, then they no longer need to compete against each other. In this way, teams or groups can begin to achieve more – what has been called synergy, something that is more than the sum total of that produced by individuals."

R Think of an alliance or inter-agency group or project of which you have been a part. Were there any partners who questioned their participation? What did each of the partners bring to the alliance?

R

Belbin's research into the working of teams (Belbin, 1981) has been extremely influential in understanding the particular problems which may arise in groups and how the contribution of individuals can be enhanced. Belbin identified eight roles which together create a balanced high performing group:

- Leader (the co-ordinator)
- Task leader (the shaper)
- Ideas person (the plant)
- Analyst (the monitor/evaluator)
- Practical organizer (company worker)
- Fix it (the resource investigator)
- Mediator (the team worker)
- Details person (the finisher)

Can you identify the role you normally play in groups?

Davies *et al.* (1993) identify a key role in alliances for the mediator, who can resolve conflicts through bargaining and exchange. They also identify a role for "the reticulist" – someone who plays a bridging role, spanning organizational boundaries and who can harness energies and skills. It is often necessary for a formally appointed co-ordinator to take on this bridging role.

Tuckman's model of group development (Tuckman, 1965) has been influential in showing how groups have common characteristics in their development. Tuckman describes groups as moving through five identifiable stages:

1. **Forming** – in which a group first meets and works out the roles of members and tries to agree a task and some way of working.
2. **Storming** – in which the group becomes polarized and may form subgroups. There may be reactions to power distribution and some resistance to the task.
3. **Norming** – in which the group begins to establish some shared goals and to find a way of working. Members take on roles to support the group in its task or to help the group work well together.
4. **Performing** – in which the group begins to work well. There is more trust and acceptance of the contribution of each member. Interpersonal issues get resolved. Members approach the task with energy.
5. **Mourning** – the group disbands, sometimes reluctantly and there may be attempts to continue the life of the group.

In the initial stages of alliance work, there may be competition (the storming phase) as the balance of power within the group is worked out. For a group to move on, however, a safe enough environment has to be created.

> **R** Think of a group or alliance of which you have been a part. Can you identify stages in the "life" of the group or alliance? What helped to move the group through the stages or did it get stuck?

In healthy alliance work, participants often focus on the task for which they have come together. Difficulties arise over the nature of the task and the role of the participating agencies in the alliance. What often gets ignored in alliance work is the "maintenance" of the alliance – those ways of being which help people to work together. Markwell (1995) for example, identifies the importance of making sure that participants are acquainted. The motivation of someone drafted in or someone who has little influence or knowledge of the echelons of their own agency may be limited. So effort in communicating about the work and keeping participants on board is vital. Having a task focus with equal opportunities for contribution and responsibility through, for example, the setting of the criteria for the alliance and chairing meetings, can help to defuse power conflicts. Conventional ways of working, such as committees, steering groups and formal minute taking can hamper the development of ideas and inhibit the contribution of community representatives who may be unused to such ways of working. Many studies of collaborative working suggest that informal arrangements can be more productive and co-operative (Delaney, 1994b; Springett, 1995).

Beattie (1994:119) argues that groups also need to develop the ability to give feedback on how the group is working. He argues that there is a strong case for drawing on "the theory and practice of

D The Department of Health (1996) produced guidance on setting up alliance work which is reproduced in Table 8.3. Does this advice indicate an understanding of theories of inter-sectoral collaboration? Are there any issues you would add?

psychodynamics of relationships within institutions to explore the significance of emotional processes and interpersonal defence mechanisms". Members need to spend time talking over differences and reviewing relationships within the alliance. Funnel *et al.* (1995) also cite communication underpinned by "simplicity, honesty and openness" as a key characteristic of an effective healthy alliance.

This section has looked at organizational and interpersonal issues drawing on established theories from management and organizational studies and social psychology and psychodynamic work. These ideas help us to make sense of those factors, identified from empirical studies, which are the ingredients for successful collaboration. The insights gained from practice can also help us to "test" these theories to see if they do offer explanations of what goes on in collaborative and alliance work.

Table 8.3 *The stages of setting up healthy alliances*

Establish Partnerships and alliances
- Identify key organizations/allies
- Agree a process for communication and co-ordination
- Agree resources
- Contact existing alliances to avoid duplication

Agree Priorities
- Jointly agree common aims, goals and priorities
- Set an agenda
- Identify a lead agency for each priority area
- Set up a healthy alliance for each area
- Identify appropriate representation
- Obtain commitment to the process and the tasks
- Clarify how to ensure that agreed work is done

Assess Needs
- Identify existing resources, information, projects (local audit of health action)
- Develop a local health profile combining health authority Annual reports with existing community information
- Agree process for needs assessment across all agencies including the public
- Consider local policies, strategies or guidelines as appropriate

Agree aims and objectives, set targets
- Review needs assessment and agree aims, objectives and targets
- Agree defined tasks for each partner
- Develop programmes in the light of existing resources

Measure Progress
- Agree between partners how to measure success
- Review aims, objectives and targets against achievements/evaluation
- Assess costs against outcomes
- Reassess priorities, aims, objectives, targets and programmes

Source: DoH (1996). Reproduced with permission

Conclusion

The theoretical frameworks and variety of experience which characterize collaboration for health reveal a number of common themes concerning the difficulties and opportunities for successful collaboration. There are obvious costs and benefits involved. Intersectoral collaboration is about compromise and entails some change in normal patterns of working. It means relinquishing control and the inclination to put one's own interests first and it entails crossing professional boundaries. It is very expensive in terms of time and resources and so it must have top level commitment. On the other hand, at the level of a specific project or campaign, intersectoral collaboration may lead to synergistic working with the achievement of more significant and long-term outcomes than would be achieved by agencies working in isolation. It may have a "trickle down" effect whereby partner agencies become more committed to health promotion and gain new insights into problem definitions and possible solutions. Intersectoral collaboration offers the potential of more "transparent" ways of working, with greater accountability to a variety of interest groups. Most fundamental of all, however, is that intersectoral collaboration can bring about a cultural change that recognizes health as a multidimensional concept not merely confined to health services.

Activity *What is a healthy alliance?*	Funnel *et al.* (1995) have set out evaluative criteria for alliances based on the "Health For All" principles of equity, collaboration and participation. The embracing of these core values will lead alliances to have certain key characteristics against which their working can be evaluated. Using the lead questions in Table 8.4, decide if an alliance in which you are a partner can be deemed "healthy".

Table 8.4 *Evaluating healthy alliances*

Commitment
1. Are there joint aims?
2. Is it clear what each partner brings to the alliance and what each can gain from it?
3. Is there senior level commitment?
   Do people attend meetings? Is non-attendance discussed?
   Do people have time for meetings? Is it in their job description?
   Do the same people attend?
4. Is the alliance balanced with public, private and voluntary sectors?
5. Is there a co-ordinator? If not, would this help?
6. How do you ensure that members have the skills and training for joint working?
7. Are new members attracted? How?
8. How do you ensure the alliance has an adequate budget?

(continued)

Table 8.4 *Evaluating healthy alliances – contd*	**Community involvement**
	9. How is the community involved?
	     Are there community members? Who?
	10. How are their views incorporated?
	11. Is there training and support for community participants?
	12. Do the community feel they have ownership?
	
	Communication
	13. Does the alliance share information?
	14. Are there reports of meetings? To whom are these distributed?
	15. Is there an agreed mechanism for feedback to organizations?
	16. Is there a corporate identity for the alliance (logo, name)?
	17. Is the alliance visible?
	
	Joint strategies
	18. Are there joint priorities, strategies, action plans?
	     How do these relate to members' other priorities in their own organizations?
	19. Do members have agreed roles?
	20. How does the alliance generate new projects?
	
	Accountability
	21. How is the alliance answerable to community and organizations?
	22. How does the alliance evaluate itself?

Adapted from Funnel et al. (1995), with permission

Further discussion

■ How do the concepts of healthy alliances and intersectoral collaboration differ?

■ Is the commitment to healthy alliances by the NHS more rhetoric than reality?

Recommended reading

■ Davies J, Dooris M, Russell J and Pettersson G (1993) *Healthy Alliances: a study of interagency collaboration in health promotion*, London, London Research Centre report for SW Thames Regional Health Authority.
This report provides a theoretical analysis of collaboration and some case studies including one on a child safety equipment scheme.

■ Delaney F (1994) "Muddling through the middle ground: theoretical concerns in intersectoral collaboration and health promotion", *Health Promotion International*, **9**(3), 217–25.
Delaney F (1994) "Making connections: research into intersectoral collaboration", *Health Education Journal*, **53**, 474–85.

These two articles discuss some of the problems and areas for development in understanding the theory of collaboration in health promotion.

- Draper P (ed.) (1991) *Health Through Public Policy*, London, Greenprint.
  Contributions on actions that could be taken to promote health and protect the environment.

- Funnel R, Oldfield K and Speller V (1995) *Towards Healthier Alliances*, London, Health Education Authority.
  Guidelines on evaluating alliances and how partners can monitor progress.

- Leathard A (ed.) (1994) *Going interprofessional: working together for health and welfare*, London, Routledge.
  An edited collection which explores the theory of interprofessional work, the rationale for interprofessional training and some examples of collaboration in child protection work, in mental healthcare and work with older people.

- Springett J (1995) *Intersectoral collaboration: Theory and Practice*, Liverpool, Institute of Health, John Moores University.
  An academic study of the theory of Intersectoral Collaboration.

- West MA and Slater J (1996) *Team working in Primary Health Care*, London, Health Education Authority.
  A report which summarizes the evidence on the effectiveness of team working and looks at the implications for multidisciplinary working in primary care.

References

Ashton J (1986) "Healthy Cities – WHO's New Public Health Initiative", *Health promotion*, **1**(3), 319–24.

Ashton J and Seymour H (1988) *The New Public Health*, Buckingham, Open University Press.

Ashton L (1995) "Ageing well: promoting the health of older people through partnership arrangements", *Conference paper Healthy Alliances in theory and practice*, Bath, Bath College of Higher Education, September 1995.

Beattie A (1994) "Healthy alliances or dangerous liaisons? The challenge of working together in health promotion", in Leathard A (ed.) *Going Interprofessional: working together for health and welfare*, London, Routledge.

Belbin RM (1981) *Management teams: why they succeed or fail*, Oxford, Butterworth Heinemann.

Benzeval M, Judge K and Whitehead M (1995) *Tackling inequalities in health*, London, Kings Fund.

Birchall E and Hallett C (1992) *Coordination of child protection*, London, HMSO.

Bloxham S (1996) "A case study of inter-agency collaboration in the education and promotion of young people's sexual health", *Health Education Journal*, **55**, 389–403.

Crombie H (1996) *Sustainable Development and Health*, Birmingham, Public Health Alliance.

Davies J, Dooris M, Russell J and Pettersson G (1993) *Healthy alliances: a study of inter-agency collaboration in health promotion*, London, London Research Centre report for South West Thames Regional Health Authority.

Delaney F (1994a) "Muddling through the middle

ground: theoretical concerns in intersectoral collaboration and health promotion", *Health Promotion International*, **9**(3), 217–25.

Delaney F (1994b) "Making connections: research into intersectoral collaboration", *Health Education Journal*, **53**, 474–85.

Department of Health (1991) *Working Together: a guide to arrangements for inter-agency cooperation for the protection of children from abuse*, London, HMSO.

Department of Health (1993) *Working Together for better health*, London, HMSO.

Department of Health (1996) *The Health of the Nation on Environmental Health*, London, HMSO.

Ewles L (1993) "Hope Against Hype", *Health Service Journal*, 26 August, pp. 30–31.

Ewles L (1996) "The impact of the NHS reforms on specialist health promotion in the NHS", in Scriven J and Orme J (eds) *Health Promotion: Professional Perspectives*, Buckingham, Open University.

Farrant W (1986) "Health For All by the year 2000?", *Radical Community Medicine*, Winter 1986/7, 19–26.

Fieldgrass J (1992) *Partnerships in health promotion*, London, Health Education Authority.

Funnel R, Oldfield K and Speller V (1995) *Towards healthier alliances*, London, Health Education Authority.

Glover M (1996) "Alliances for health at work: a case study", in Scriven A and Orme J (eds) *Health Promotion: Professional Perspectives*, Buckingham, Open University.

Hancock T (1993) "Health, human development and the community ecosystem: three ecological models", *Health Promotion International*, **8**(1), 41–46.

Handy C (1976) *Understanding organizations*, London, Penguin.

Hogg C (1991) *Healthy Change*, London, Socialist Health Association.

Hudson B (1987) "Collaboration in social welfare", *Policy and politics*, **15**, 175–82.

Institute of Health Service Managers (1990) *Health For All Questionnaire – revised evaluation*, IHSM.

Labonte R (1991) "Econology: integrating health and sustainable development", *Health Promotion International*, **6**(1), 49–65.

Leathard A (1994) (ed.) *Going interprofessional:*

working together for health and welfare, London, Routledge.

Markwell S (1995) "Exploration of conflict theory within healthy alliances", *Conference paper Healthy Alliances in theory and Practice*, Bath, Bath College of Higher Education, September 1995.

Nutbeam D (1994) "Intersectoral action for health: making it work", *Health Promotion International*, **9**(3), 143–44.

Ovreteit J (1993) *Coordinating community care: multidisciplinary teams and care management*, Buckingham, Open University Press.

Powell M (1992) *Healthy alliances: report to the Health Gain Standing Conference*, London, Office of Public Management.

Scambler G and Goraya A (1994) "Movements for change: the new public health agenda", *Critical Public Health*, **5**(2), 4–9.

Scott Samuel A (1996) "Health Impact Assessment", *Public Health Alliance News*, Summer.

Scriven A (1995) "Healthy alliances: the results of a national audit", *Health Education Journal*, **54**, 176–85.

Simnett I (1995) *Managing health promotion: developing healthy organisations and communities*, Chichester, Wiley.

Springett J (1995) *Intersectoral Collaboration: theory and practice*, Liverpool, Institute for Health, John Moores University.

Thomas C (1993) "Public health strategies in Sheffield and England: a comparison of conceptual foundations", *Health Promotion International*, **8**(4), 299–307.

Townsend P and Davidson N (1982) *Inequalities in health: The Black Report*, London, Penguin.

Tuckman BW (1965) "Developmental sequence in small groups", *Psychological Bulletin*, **63**, 384–99.

West MA and Slater J (1996) *Team Working in Primary Health Care*, London, Health Education Authority.

WHO (1978) *Alma Ata 1978 Primary Health Care*, Copenhagen, WHO.

WHO (1985) *Health for All in Europe by the Year 2000*, Copenhagen, WHO.

WHO (1986) *Ottawa Charter for Health Promotion: an international conference on health promotion*, Geneva, WHO.

WHO (1988) *Adelaide Recommendations on Healthy Public Policy*, Adelaide, WHO.

PART 3

Challenges in Practice

Introduction

This section examines five key issues which were identified in the "Health of the Nation" strategy (DoH, 1992) and which will remain priorities for health promotion. The issues selected met three criteria: the key areas represented a large burden of preventable disease and premature death; evidence existed of effective interventions which could reduce this toll of ill-health and premature death; and it was possible to set targets and monitor progress.

This disease focus has been widely criticized for ignoring the pre-requisites of health such as adequate income, housing and employment prospects (Brown and Piper, 1997; Smith, 1991; Radical Statistics Health Group, 1991). The new Labour government has acknowledged these limitations and declared its intention to build on existing strategies but at the same time to move beyond lifestyle risk factors and a focus on diseases to address social economic and environmental factors and the needs of particular population groups such as children and older people (DoH, 1997).

Despite criticisms, the introduction of the "Health of the Nation" strategy in 1992 was welcomed for focusing on health in a planned way. The existence of national key areas and targets acted as a spur to practitioners and policy makers, presenting many new opportunities. This section includes case studies to illustrate some examples of innovative interventions and some examples where pursuing the core principles of health promotion has proved difficult.

Each chapter in this section reports on a key area, and benefits from the co-authorship of practitioners from the field who are best placed to identify what has informed the development of particular interventions, as well as the barriers which need to be addressed in order to promote effective interventions. The views expressed reflect the individual views of different practitioners, which in turn reflect the diversity of opinion within the field.

There are some important differences between the key issues. Cardiovascular disease and cancers are disease conditions which are known to be related to certain risk factors, some of which are modifiable by individual behaviour change. The key debates surrounding these areas are the nature of identified risk factors and how these may be affected. The two chapters on cardiovascular disease and cancers provide an overview of the range of strategies adopted in a particular locality.

By contrast, for the key areas of mental and sexual health there are immediate problems of definition. These terms are the subject of much debate, and the two chapters examining these areas adopt a more critical approach, examining at the outset problems of definition. They do not seek to present a comprehensive overview, but instead seek to explore the territory in the light of existing practice.

The key area of accidents straddles these boundaries, being both a disease category in medical statistics but also an area where the central notion of risk is debated and contested. The chapter on accidents provides a critical review of some accident prevention interventions.

References

Brown PA and Piper SM (1997) "Nursing and the health of the nation: Schism or symbiosis," *Journal of Advanced Nursing*, **25**, 297–301.

Department of Health (1992) *The Health of the Nation: A strategy for health in England*, London, HMSO.

Department of Health (1997) *Target: Our Healthier Nation*, London, Department of Health.

Radical Statistics Health Group (1991) "Missing: A strategy for health of the nation", *British Medical Journal*, **303**, 299–302.

Smith T (1990) "Poverty and health in the 1990s", *British Medical Journal*, **301**, 349–350.

9 *Reducing accidents*

Jeremy Cole, Jennie Naidoo and Jane Wills

Key points

- National strategy on accident reduction.
- Epidemiological and lay risk assessment.
- Accident reduction strategies incorporating:
- Equity, participation, empowerment, inter-agency working.

Overview

This chapter discusses the way in which strategies to reduce accidents are constructed. It argues that government policy sees accidents as avoidable events which are the consequence of individual behaviour and can thus be prevented through safety education. However the evidence is that legislation and technical safety measures are more likely to be effective. The chapter looks at two projects – a home safety equipment loan scheme and a project which links information from accident sites with hospital information on injury levels. Both projects show how health promotion has moved beyond its traditional educational role to address the structural causes of accidents. These examples of practice illustrate the potential for intersectoral and interdepartmental co-ordination of policy. The chapter concludes that although reducing accidents is a huge task which may seem beyond the role of individual health promoters, innovative practice is possible which strikes a balance between realism and fundamental principles of health promotion.

Introduction

Accidents are the commonest cause of death among people under 30 in England and Wales, although the absolute number of deaths is greatest in people aged 65 and over (OPCS, 1991). Accidents are also a major cause of injury and disability and a considerable burden on the health and emergency services. Accidents represent one of the greatest public health problems. The "Health of the Nation" strategy set targets for reducing the mortality rate for children under 15 (by at least 33%), young people aged 15–24 (by at least 25%) and for people over 65 years (by at least 33%).

Risk has become the critical, determining concept in constructing strategies aimed at reducing accidental injury. As epidemiology

D The basis of the national strategy on accidents is that they are predictable and therefore preventable. Do you agree?

reveals that certain factors are associated with an increased risk of accidental injury, so preventive activity addresses itself to removing or controlling those risk factors. However, while the epidemiology of accidents can be mapped and, at a population level, planned interventions can certainly reduce rates of accidental injury, general statistical tendencies conceal a chaotic distribution of accidents. Risk factors can never tell us where and when or whom a particular accident will strike. As a unique event, an accident remains unpredictable (Green, 1995) and, by implication, unavoidable.

As we saw in Chapter 5, there can be a tension then between lay and scientific concepts of risk. Reductions in accident rates are visible to an epidemiologist but, to the ordinary citizen, accidents avoided in a population are simply events that never took place. The people unwittingly spared are faceless and nameless. In life, an accident prevented is not an accident, and an accident that occurs cannot be prevented (Cole, 1995:61). The epidemiological concept of risk, from which priorities for prevention are derived, belongs not in the real world but in the world of mathematical probability (Davison *et al.*, 1992:108).

While epidemiological analysis has led to accident reduction becoming a priority area, health promotion seeks to tackle accidents according to fundamental principles of equity, empowerment and participation. This chapter explores some of the resulting dilemmas and presents case studies to illustrate innovative practice in this area.

Accident prevention

Over the last 30 years, England has seen an overall downward trend in accidental deaths which can probably be attributed to successful measures already taken to prevent accidents and to advances in emergency medical care in hospitals and at the scene of accidents. Nevertheless, accidents remain a significant public health problem, accounting for over 10,000 deaths a year in England (OPCS, 1991) and 7% of total NHS expenditure (DoH, 1992). Because of a relative lack of morbidity data, the injury and disability caused by accidents are more difficult to quantify.

Accidents in childhood

Among children, the mortality rate for accidents has declined more slowly than the mortality rate for other causes (Milner, 1995) and accidents are now exposed as by far the leading cause of death in children over the age of one. In the UK, over 600 children under 15 died as a result of accidents in 1993 (Hogg, 1996). It is estimated that each year unintentional injury in this age group affects the long-term health of some 10,000 children (DoH, 1993) and costs the NHS £200 million (CAPT, 1992).

Accidents among young adults

In the 15–24 year age group, 1234 people were killed in accidents in 1991 (OPCS, 1991). Almost half of all deaths in 15–19 year olds and more than a third of deaths in 20–24 year olds resulted from accidents. Moreover, the general downward trend in accident mortality appears to have halted in this age group (DoH, 1993).

Accidents among older people

Among people aged 65 and over, accidents are not a major cause of death compared with other causes. But, while they account for only a relatively small proportion of deaths, the mortality rate for accidents is actually highest in this age group. In 1991, 4626 people over 64 died as a result of accidents (OPCS, 1991). Falls account for the majority of accidents among people over 64. With the consequences of falling becoming more severe with advancing age, demographic projections of a relative increase in the number of people over 75 in the population suggest that the problem will worsen in years to come (FPSC, 1994).

International literature reviews have considered the effectiveness of interventions to reduce different types of accident among children and young adults (Towner *et al.*, 1993; Munro *et al.*, 1995; NHS Centre for Reviews and Dissemination, 1996a) and to prevent falls and subsequent injury among older people (NHS Centre for Reviews and Dissemination, 1996b). The quantity of studies reviewed and the heterogeneity of accidents, both between and within age groups, prevent synthesis of the results here. As a general point though, it was found that few interventions in any age group had been evaluated rigorously enough to conclude beyond all doubt that they were effective in reducing accidental death or injury. Even so, taking the evidence as a whole, it is possible to make some general observations about the effectiveness of accident prevention interventions. (The general issue of effectiveness and evidence-based practice is discussed further in Chapter 3.)

The three Es of accident prevention

Conventionally, accident prevention activities are categorized as education, engineering or enforcement:

- **Education** involves raising awareness of hazards and how to avoid them. Examples include Junior Citizen schemes, Traffic Clubs and mass media campaigns as well as more traditional methods of imparting advice and information, such as leaflets, posters and safety counselling.
- **Engineering** refers to technical measures to increase the safety of the environment. For example, the provision of cycle paths

and pedestrian crossings, child-resistant packaging of medicines, smoke alarms in social housing, air-bags in cars.

- ■ **Enforcement** is the use of legislation, regulations and standards to reduce accidents or control injury. For example, the compulsory wearing of seat-belts or motorcycle helmets, compliance with building regulations, product-testing for conformity with safety standards.

The common theme to emerge from the literature reviews is that engineering and enforcement can be effective, but that educational interventions alone are unlikely to succeed. However, when used alongside a range of other methods, education may foster a climate of public opinion receptive to the idea of legal or environmental action. Community safety programmes, which are characterized by multi-agency working and community participation, have adopted this approach and shown some promise in simultaneously reducing injury or the risk of injury from a variety of causes (e.g. Schelp, 1987; Guyer *et al.*, 1989).

For many commentators the failure of isolated educational interventions is explained by the social and political context of accidents (e.g. Pless, 1995). A child from social class V is four times as likely to suffer a fatal accident as a child from social class I (DoH, 1996), with the children of unemployed single mothers having the worst death rates of all (Roberts and Pless, 1995).

D	How do you account for the pronounced inverse relationship between the accident mortality rate in childhood and social class? What health promotion interventions might be effective in reducing childhood accidents?

The relative inability of children to master hazardous environments might explain why they seem more susceptible than adults to the effects of structural inequality. For example, a key determinant of injuries to child pedestrians is the number of roads they cross and children of families in the lowest quarter of income cross 50% more roads than those of families in the highest quarter (Roberts *et al.*, 1994). Consistent with this is the finding that a family's lack of access to a car is associated with a doubling of the risk of childhood pedestrian injury (Roberts *et al.*, 1995).

Activity	The clear associations between elevated accident rates and social and material disadvantage suggest that social policy can have a powerful effect on accident rates. The following have been suggested as social policy interventions with the potential to reduce accidents. How might they do this? What other policy interventions can you think of?

- Subsidizing public transport.
- Increasing social welfare benefits.
- Upgrading stocks of social housing.
- More comprehensive nursery provision.

Health promotion strategies to reduce accidents

The view that health promotion methods are largely the product of ideology is supported by the persistence of accident reduction strategies that derive from professional authority and focus on individual behaviour change. Examples include traditional education as well as advice and information in the form of leaflets and posters. Mass media campaigns are also included. Although they have a mass audience, any behavioural outcomes depend on people's individual responses to the message. Since there is scant evidence that any of these methods work (Towner *et al.*, 1993; Munro *et al.*, 1995; NHS Centre for Reviews and Dissemination, 1996a, 1996b) their continued popularity is only explicable in other terms.

Implicit in such methods is the ideological assumption that the avoidance of accidents is a matter of personal responsibility and individual free choice. Conservative government policy was constructed upon this libertarian ideology and consequently sought to limit state interference in the way people choose to lead their lives. The "Health of the Nation" strategy thus stated that "the Government will rely primarily on information and education (as its preferred preventive strategies) and will avoid the imposition of unnecessary regulations on business and individuals" (DoH, 1992:106).

This ideological standpoint is at odds with the more collectivist tendencies that have dominated academic thinking in the field of health promotion in recent years and which locate the causes of accidents deep within the structures of society (e.g. McDowell, 1996). Naidoo's (1986) criticism of the 1981 Play it Safe! television campaign is typical. By holding individuals responsible for their own safety, she reasons that individually-focused initiatives are, in effect, blaming the victims of accidents for their own predicament.

Beattie (1991:169) offers an alternative explanation for the enduring popularity of what he calls health persuasion tactics. Part of their appeal to policy makers, he argues, is that they are highly visible yet at the same time simple to plan and relatively cheap to implement, requiring no more than the identification of predisposing factors for accidental injury and their communication to the population at risk.

As the case for health persuasion techniques has become increasingly discredited in health promotion circles, so has support grown for legislative and environmental action to reduce accidents, particularly from within the burgeoning "new public health" movement.

The World Health Organization's (WHO) "Targets for Health for All" challenges member states to use legislative, administrative and economic mechanisms to tackle a wide range of health issues, including accidents (WHO, 1985). The Ottawa Charter for Health Promotion (WHO, 1986) further reinforces the idea that health cannot be understood in isolation from social conditions and urges action to ensure safe products, public services and environments.

Activity

Which of the following would you regard as acceptable measures to reduce accidents?

- Random breath-testing of road users.
- Cycle helmets made compulsory for child cyclists.
- Cycle helmets made compulsory for all cyclists.
- All electrical appliances supplied with a plug fitted.
- A 20 m.p.h. speed limit in residential areas.
- Lockable windows on and above the first floor of domestic premises.
- Dual air-bags fitted to all new cars.
- Integral mains-wired smoke alarms in all domestic premises.
- A driving test for all motorists when they reach 70 years old.

Legislative action for health is associated with "old left" reformism, characterized by a paternalistic political philosophy concerned with the recuperation of social injustices (Beattie, 1991). Naidoo and Wills (1994:130) point out that social policy and legislative interventions can equally be employed within right wing ideologies, provided pursuit of the common good does not excessively curtail individual freedom.

Collective authoritarian methods have been used successfully to prevent accidents and mitigate injury. Traffic calming schemes, remedial highway engineering, the child-resistant packaging of drugs, the compulsory use of seat-belts in cars and of helmets on motorcycles have all proved effective in reducing accidental death or injury (Sabey, 1980; Towner et al., 1993). However, health promoters in the NHS have an equivocal role in public health measures of this kind; they have very little direct influence over the safety of people's environments and lobbying is unlikely to bring about changes in social policy which are inconsistent with the prevailing political ethos.

At a local level, responsibility for the safety of our living, working and travelling environments rests chiefly with the Health and Safety Executive (HSE), the police and various local authority departments; highways, housing, environmental health. The health service has been encouraged to forge alliances with these groups. By supplying information on the incidence, causes, severity and cost of accidents, the aim is to co-ordinate joint strategies that make the most effective use of combined resources to address national targets and local priorities. However, in practice, partner organizations may be unable or unwilling to redeploy resources in this way. For example, the enforcement of Health and Safety at Work remains a statutory responsibility of local authorities and the HSE even though people of working age were almost entirely excluded from the "Health of the Nation" target groups.

The dominance of epidemiological risk factors in guiding accident prevention work has left little room for methods that empower individuals or groups to play an active part in determining and responding to their own priorities. However, Community Development holds for some health promoters the promise of addressing the structural factors associated with poor health and accidents, while avoiding the accusations of collectivist paternalism sometimes levelled at traditional public health strategies (e.g. Garside, 1987).

In reality, workers who favour this method face a number of difficulties and there are few cases where community development has been used as means of accident prevention. Some large-scale community safety programmes have involved or consulted with the target community, but generally their goal seems to be winning support for the professional agenda rather than identifying or addressing local people's concerns. On a smaller scale, occasional examples can be found of neighbourhood projects taking an approach that supports local residents in deciding their own accident prevention priorities and which advertises itself as community development (e.g. Blackburn, 1991). But, while the developmental process does seem to confer certain benefits in terms of increased confidence and a sense of empowerment in participating communities, whether or not it prevents accidents is unknown. In a climate where target-effectiveness and evidence-based practice are the watchwords, the funding problems already faced by community development projects (Naidoo and Wills, 1994:171) are likely to be exacerbated.

The case for community development is further complicated by internal contradictions. First is the potential dilemma faced by community development workers in resolving conflicts between community and managerial expectations, especially when the project has been set up to tackle a single, predetermined issue such as accidents. Second, it is a paradox that professionals decide where and when to adopt a community development approach, as though it were a special prescription reserved for at-risk groups.

In summary, it has been shown that the adoption of a particular accident prevention strategy does not depend simply on evidence for its effectiveness in a given situation.

R What other factors might influence the adoption of particular strategies to reduce accidents?

C ase study

The Eastbourne Child Safety Equipment Loan Scheme

Home safety equipment schemes have grown in popularity since they first appeared in the 1980s and are nowadays held up as examples of good practice in joint working (Hogg, 1996). They may be run in a number of ways depending on local circumstances and available funding, but the common purpose is to supply families with items of child safety equipment either free of charge or at a reduced cost. Sometimes the equipment is loaned and sometimes it is given away or sold cheaply. This case study analyses the Eastbourne Child Safety Equipment Loan Scheme, although many of the observations are applicable to similar projects.

The Eastbourne scheme was launched in 1994 as a joint project between Eastbourne Borough Council and the local health authority, with families referred to the scheme by their health visitor. To qualify to borrow equipment, applicants should normally be in receipt of state benefits. Large items of equipment are loaned free of charge until the youngest child in the family reaches four years old in the case of stairgates, or five years old in the case of fireguards. Smaller items are not expected to be returned. The equipment is delivered by a council employee who will also carry out installations at the client's request. The scheme supplies around 350 families a year within a total annual budget of about £17,000, which includes the purchase of equipment, administration, transport, wages and employers' on-costs. The expense of buying new equipment is projected to diminish as more items become due for return. A process evaluation found that the scheme was rated very highly by clients and health workers alike.

To what extent does this scheme tackle social inequalities in childhood accidents? The scheme targets those on low incomes and in receipt of benefit. Is targeting in this way justifiable? Stigmatizing?

On the face of it, a home safety equipment scheme can be targeted to address inequalities in childhood accident rates and appears to avoid the charges of victim-blaming often levelled at educational and awareness-raising interventions.

In Eastbourne, the community was not consulted about the need for a scheme nor about the items of equipment that would be offered. Both these decisions were taken by professionals on the basis of accident statistics and product tests on the various types of child safety equipment on the market (DTI, 1991). The loan scheme therefore stems from the authority of local government and the NHS and has as its collective focus low-income families with young children.

The principle of community participation in service planning is enshrined in the Declaration of Alma Ata (WHO, 1978), yet the reasons for failure to consult are practical ones, encountered daily by health promoters. Half the funding for the Eastbourne scheme was from a small allocation set aside annually for "Health of the Nation" projects. The conditions for obtaining a grant required the proposal of a concrete project that addressed one of those areas identified in the "Health of the Nation", initially within one year. Exercises in public needs assessment do not meet these criteria and are not eligible for funds. If public views had been sought, they might have identified issues outside the "Health of the Nation" priorities, which could not therefore have been acted upon. Even if a loan scheme had emerged as the community's priority, its stock of equipment was not negotiable. The project co-ordinators did not feel able to supply anything that was not associated with reduced accident risk, far less anything that was potentially hazardous, for example cooker guards (DTI, 1991). To have consulted on this matter would simply have been an exercise in securing public support for a predetermined professional agenda. Either way, without the ability to respond to whatever needs the community might express, public consultation is, at best, a wasteful rigmarole and, at worst, a dishonest charade.

Most commentators in the field of healthcare ethics agree that targeting is justifiable if it works to the advantage of the least well off (Gillon, 1985:90). Nevertheless, the targeting of health promotion is not without complications, as was discussed in Chapter 5. In the field of accident prevention, the elevated death and injury rates found among children of families in lower socio-economic groups are frequently attributed to parental fecklessness or working class fatalism (Avery and Jackson, 1993:12–13), although there is little support for either phenomenon in the literature (Cole, 1995). It is also worth reiterating that the epidemiological concept of risk is only concerned with mathematical probabilities and disguises the haphazard distribution of accidents in a population. This is sometimes forgotten. The result is that low-income families suffer from a general "at-risk" label while accidents are not seen as an issue for wealthier families.

Targeting creates operational as well as ethical difficulties. On the one hand, Eastbourne council argued for hard and fast criteria for eligibility to the loan scheme, namely that applicants should be in receipt of income support or family credit. Several health visitors, on the other hand, felt that the central issue was the protection of children, regardless of their parents' income and that safety equipment should be lent at their discretion to families who would not provide it themselves, as well as to those who could not. Health visitors were also reluctant to become involved in means-testing, arguing that their relationship with clients would be undermined if they were viewed as agents of the benefits system.

A compromise was reached to regard the conditions for eligibility as guidelines rather than binding rules. Although health visitors can now exercise some discretion when making referrals to the scheme, they are still advised to consider exceptions carefully since they might find themselves in an invidious position if the system is believed to be working arbitrarily. Furthermore, clients declare themselves in receipt of benefit and do not have to produce evidence for inspection by their health visitor.

McDowell (1996:5) criticizes local home safety equipment schemes as peripheral to the deep-seated structural causes of childhood accidents and urges instead the universal provision of equipment though the welfare benefits system. However, it has already been argued that calls for far-reaching changes in social policy are unlikely to be heeded in the prevailing political climate. The choice for health promoters is either to whistle in the wind or to take action that strikes a balance between principles and practicality.

The following case study illustrates the potential and problems of a "Healthy Alliance" approach to accident reduction.

Case study

Injury prevention through data linkage

This case study examines a multi-agency pilot project which has found a potential role for the health service in the planning of environmental safety measures. The East Sussex Accident Prevention Group was convened by the local health authority as a "healthy alliance" (DoH, 1993:53). The health authority is represented by its health promotion, public health and information departments. Also represented are the highways, education and road safety departments of the county council, the Health and Safety Executive, local authorities, the emergency services and the South East Institute of Public Health, a division of the United Medical and Dental Schools of Guy's and St Thomas' Hospitals which undertakes research and consultancy work for a variety of public sector clients. Constraints on the funding of all member organizations precluded large-scale expenditure on new projects and have focused the group's attention instead on making more effective use of existing resources.

Road accidents are a major cause of accidental death and injury across the age range. Nationally, highways departments and the police have a target of reducing road casualties by one third by 2000. This target was set by the Department of Transport (DoT) in 1987 and takes as its baseline the annual average of road casualties in the years 1981 to 1985 (DoT, 1987). Before-and-after studies at sites with a high incidence of road accidents (or accident "blackspots" as they are commonly known) have shown that remedial highway engineering measures consistently result in a very rapid return on investment in terms of casualty savings (Mackie, 1996). Indeed, highway engineering is held to be among the most cost-effective of public health interventions (Graham and Vaupel, 1981).

The priority for highway engineers is sites with the worst records for accidents coded by the police as fatal and serious. Current coding rules dictate that any road accident resulting in admission to hospital is classified in one of these two categories. The "serious" classification is the same whether the casualty is admitted for a single night's observation or suffers permanent disability. Although police reports only have this very limited detail of any injuries sustained, they do contain a wealth of material about the circumstances of a road accident. In contrast, hospital in-patient data describe fully the treatment given to a casualty and the outcome, but provide no information about cause, other than that a road accident was involved. Consequently, it is not possible to determine which road accidents cause the worst injuries.

The aim of the data linkage pilot project was to match police road accident reports with hospital inpatient cases. A linked database was expected to provide a clearer overall picture of road accidents, allowing partner agencies in the Accident Prevention Group to target road safety interventions more effectively and, in particular, to enable highway engineers to prioritize for remedial works the sites of "serious" accidents leading to the most severe and costly injury outcomes.

The South East Institute of Public Health was commissioned by the Accident Prevention Group to conduct the pilot project, which linked data on casualties admitted to hospitals in Eastbourne and Hastings with police road accident reports. The project was funded by a grant of £7800 from the regional health authority. The result of the pilot project was the successful linking of 77% of cases, with potential for greater linkage performance in future. It also uncovered inaccuracies in police data and identified the most cost-effective linkage method (Cryer, Brunning and Rahman, 1995).

Both the local highways department and the health authority are keen to employ a linked database for determining future engineering priorities, giving greatest weight to those accidents which result in the most severe injury. However, there is a need to retain the current coding system (i.e. fatal, serious, slight) which is used nationally because it permits comparison between the performance of different districts. One highways department cannot unilaterally adopt a new system, even if it is more sophisticated. The practical application of a linked database in road safety planning therefore depends on East Sussex successfully lobbying to become a pilot area for the new system.

This case study illustrates a tension between the national accident prevention strategies of different Government departments. The Department of Health calls on the NHS to provide other organizations with improved accident data so they can target their preventive activities more accurately, yet the Department of Transport's injury coding system prescribes how police and highways departments must target their preventive work. The same tension is further evident in the different targets for accident prevention of the two departments. Since road accidents comprise either the highest percentage or the highest actual number of accidental deaths in the three "Health of the Nation" target age groups, there is the potential for interdepartmental co-ordination of policy to establish shared targets and a joint strategy for achieving them.

At the time of writing it is still too soon to say how much influence the new appointment of a minister for public health will be able to have across Government departments, but the data linkage project shows how collaboration can synthesize the existing knowledge of separate organizations into something that exceeds the sum of its parts. It also raises interesting questions about the nature of health promotion. At first sight, few people would identify the data linkage project as health promotion. Nonetheless, if health promotion is to move beyond the much criticized and largely ineffective educational methods with which it has been associated in the past, it must seek ways of influencing the agendas of a variety of organizations; a process made easier when there is mutual benefit to be gained. In this case, the use of a linked database as a planning tool promises potential advantages to both the health service and the highways department. The health service can expect a reduction in the burden of severe injuries resulting from road accidents. The highways department can expect to quantify more accurately the returns on its investment in highway engineering. As this happens, the cost–benefits to the NHS of highway engineering will become apparent and calculable. In the longer term, this raises the tantalizing prospect of health authorities purchasing road safety measures from highways departments in just the same way as they currently purchase conventional preventive services, such as immunization or screening programmes, from more traditional health service providers.

D Taking the example of childhood accidents, identify appropriate agencies to form a healthy alliance. What benefits would accrue to each agency?

Conclusion

There is often a world of difference between the ideal of health promotion as action to optimize people's health by improving their ways and conditions of living and health promotion as practised by the self-styled health promoter. In many ways this reflects the gulf between theory and practice. Wholesale economic and social reform is beyond the power of any one individual or group, but if health promotion fails to address these influences it will remain at the margins. In the present economic climate, the future viability of health promotion depends on its ability to compete successfully for resources on a playing field that often slopes in favour of medical interventions. An ounce of prevention is expected to be not only better than a pound of cure, but cheaper as well. The challenge for health promoters is to find ways of working that strike a balance between idealism and realism, without unduly compromising the fundamental principles of health promotion. The child safety equipment loan scheme and the data linkage project demonstrate how innovative practice seeks to reconcile conflicting demands.

Further discussion

- Why might it be important to understand lay explanations for the causes of accidents? Can these be dismissed as irrational and fatalistic?
- How does the key area of accidents illustrate the importance of intersectoral and inter-agency working?

Recommended reading

- CAPT (1994) *Loan Schemes for Home Safety Equipment*, London, Child Accident Prevention Trust.
  A practical step-by-step guide on how to fund, set up, run and evaluate a home safety equipment scheme.

- Department of Health (1993) *Key Area Handbook – Accidents*, London, HMSO.
  A "Health of the Nation" handbook which explains why reducing accidents is a government priority and sets out what the NHS can do to meet its targets. The handbook includes chapters on the scale of the problem, working as part of an alliance and the problems of data collection.

- Scott S, Williams G, Platt S and Thomas H (eds) (1992) *Private Risks and Public Dangers*, Aldershot, Avebury.
  A diverse collection of challenging and stimulating chapters exploring many of the theoretical, ideological and philosophical issues at the heart of accident prevention work.

References

Beattie A (1991) "Knowledge and Control in Health Promotion: A Test Case for Social Policy and Social Theory", in Gabe J, Calnan, M and Bury, M (eds) *Sociology of the Health Service*, Chapter 7, London, Routledge and Kegan Paul.

Blackburn C (1991) "The Boxhill Parents' Group", in *Preventing Accidents to Children: A Training Resource for Health Visitors*, pp. 83–87, London, Child Accident Prevention Trust/Health Education Authority.

CAPT (1992) *The NHS and Social Costs of Children's Accidents*, London, Child Accident Prevention Trust.

Cole J (1995) *Outrageous Fortune: An Investigation of Maternal Beliefs about the Causes of Childhood Accidents and their Relationship with Attitudes towards Child Safety Equipment*, London, Unpublished MSc Dissertation, South Bank University.

Cryer C, Brunning D and Rahman M (1995) *Injury Prevention through Data Linkage. Phase 2: Data Linkage Pilot*, Tunbridge Wells, South East Institute of Public Health.

Davison C, Frankel S and Davey-Smith G (1992) "To Hell with Tomorrow: Coronary Heart Disease Risk and the Ethnography of Fatalism", in Scott S, Williams G, Platt S, Thomas H (eds) *Private Risks and Public Dangers*, Chapter 3, Aldershot, Avebury.

Department of Health (1992) *The Health of the Nation*, London, HMSO.

Department of Health (1993) *Key Area Handbook – Accidents*, London, HMSO.

Department of Health (1996) *Variations in Health: What Can the Department of Health and the NHS Do?* London, HMSO.

DTI (1991) *Child Safety Equipment for Use in the Home*, London, Department of Trade and Industry.

Department of Transport (1987) *Road Safety: The Next Steps*, London, HMSO.

FPSC (1994) *Putting Families on the Map: Factsheet 1*, London, Family Policy Studies Centre.

Garside P (1987) *History of Public Health*, Paper for Rethinking Public Health Conference, July 1987, Birmingham.

Gillon R (1985) *Philosophical Medical Ethics*, Chichester, Wiley.

Graham J and Vaupel J (1981) "Value of life: What difference does it make?" *Risk Analysis*, **1**, 89–95.

Green J (1995) "Accidents and the Risk Society: Some Problems with Prevention", in Bunton R, Nettleton S and Burrows R (eds) *The Sociology of Health Promotion*, London, Routledge.

Guyer B, Gallagher S, Chang B, Azzara C, Cupples L and Colton T (1989) "Prevention of childhood injuries: Evaluation of the Statewide Childhood Injury Prevention Program (SCIPP)", *American Journal of Public Health*, **79**, 1521–27.

Hogg C (1996) *Preventing Children's Accidents: A Guide for Health Authorities and Boards*, London, Child Accident Prevention Trust.

Mackie, A (1996) *Monitoring of Local Authority Safety Schemes*, Crowthorne, Transport Research Laboratory on behalf of the County Surveyors' Society.

McDowell O (1996) *Accident Prevention*. Unpublished draft position paper of the Society of Health Education and Promotion Specialists.

Milner D (1995) *Health of the Nation: Improving Information on Accidents*, in Child Accident Prevention Through Healthy Alliances, Conference Proceedings, June 1995, Avonsafe and Child Accident Prevention in Shropshire, London, Health Education Authority.

Munro J, Coleman P, Nichol J, Harper R, Kent G and Wild D (1995) "Can we prevent accidental injury to adolescents? A systematic review of the evidence", *Injury Prevention*, **1**, 249–55.

Naidoo J (1986) "Limits to Individualism", in Rodmell S and Watt A (eds), *The Politics of Health Education*, Chapter 2, London, Routledge and Kegan Paul.

Naidoo J and Wills J (1994) *Health Promotion: Foundations for Practice*, London, Baillière Tindall.

NHS Centre for Reviews and Dissemination (1996a) "Preventing unintentional injuries in children and young adolescents", *Effective Health Care*, **2**(5).

NHS Centre for Reviews and Dissemination (1996b) "Preventing falls and subsequent injury in older people", *Effective Health Care*, **2**(4).

Office of Population Censuses and Surveys (1991) *Mortality Statistics on Accidents and Violence*, London, HMSO.

Pless I (1995) "Logo and logic (editorial)", *Injury Prevention*, **1**(1), 1–2.

Roberts I and Pless B (1995) "Social policy as a cause of childhood accidents: The children of lone mothers", *British Medical Journal*, **311**, 925–28.

Roberts I, Keal M and Frith W J (1994) "Pedestrian exposure and the risk of child pedestrian injury", *Journal of Paediatric Child Health*, **30**, 220–23.

Roberts I, Norton R, Jackson R, Dunn, R and Hassall, I (1995) "Environmental factors and the risk of child pedestrian injury: A case-control study", *British Medical Journal*, **310**, 91–94.

Sabey B (1980) *Road Safety and Value for Money*. Transport and Road Research Laboratory supplementary report 581, TRRL, Crowthorne.

Schelp L (1987) "Community intervention and changes in accident pattern in a rural Swedish municipality", *Health Promotion*, **2**, 109–25.

Towner E, Dowswell T and Jarvis S (1993) *Reducing Childhood Accidents*, London, Health Education Authority.

WHO (1978) *Report of the International Conference on Primary Health Care*, Alma Ata, Geneva, World Health Organization.

WHO (1985) *Targets for Health for All*, Copenhagen, World Health Organization.

WHO (1986) "Ottawa Charter for Health Promotion", *Journal of Health Promotion*, **1**, i–v.

10 The prevention of coronary heart disease and stroke

Jennie Naidoo, Vicki Taylor and Jane Wills

Key points

- National health strategy and cardiovascular disease.
- Evidence of effective interventions.
- Health promotion and healthy eating.
- Health promotion and physical activity.

Overview

Cardiovascular disease (CVD) which includes coronary heart disease (CHD) and stroke is multifactorial but is often perceived as a single issue to be addressed. The focus of health promotion is on risk behaviours for CVD:

- nutrition and especially intake of saturated fats;
- smoking;
- sedentary lifestyles.

This chapter provides an overview of approaches to encouraging healthy eating and physical activity. The next chapter on cancers looks at smoking prevention and education. CVD is also affected by risk situations – adverse social and environmental conditions such as poverty or poor working and living conditions. Many risk behaviours (smoking, excessive drinking, lack of exercise) are a response to the conditions in which people live. Such conditions combine to create a level of susceptibility to this preventable disease. This chapter looks at three examples of health promotion interventions which seek to address the socio-economic factors which contribute to differential opportunities to be healthy. The St Pancras food shop illustrates how access to cheap food can be made easier for housebound older people. Health at Work in the NHS is an initiative which encourages NHS premises to make it easier for employees to adopt healthy lifestyles. Developing transport policy at a local level is a complex task requiring major intersectoral collaboration and commitment at all levels and is an example of how agencies can work together to encourage alternative forms of transport which protect the environment and encourage physical activity.

Introduction

"Coronary Heart Disease (CHD) accounted for about 26% of deaths in England in 1991. It is both the single largest cause of death, and the single main cause of premature death. It accounts for 2.5% of total NHS expenditure, and results in 35 million lost working days per year. Approximately 12% of all deaths in 1991 resulted from stroke, which is also a major cause of disability, particularly amongst elderly people. Stroke accounts for 6% of total NHS expenditure and results in the loss of about 7.7 million working days each year"

(DoH, 1992).

Reducing coronary heart disease and stroke are, thus, major priorities for health promotion. However, despite considerable research there remains a degree of uncertainty about the key risk factors for CHD and stroke. Current knowledge suggests that the most important risk factors are: cigarette smoking, blood lipids (total cholesterol/HDL cholesterol/triglycerides), raised blood pressure (hypertension) and physical inactivity. However, the relationship between fat consumption and incidence of CHD has been challenged (Le Fanu, 1991). Accepted contributory risk factors include excessive alcohol consumption, obesity, excessive salt intake and diabetes although the association between alcohol and CHD is still under discussion (data from the British Regional Heart Study in 1981 showed a strong positive correlation between alcohol and CHD on a town basis but this may be a consequence of the strong correlation between alcohol intake and cigarette smoking). Little is known about how these risk factors interact but there is agreement that in most cases multiple risk factors are implicated.

In the "Health of the Nation" strategy for CHD and stroke in 1993 (DoH, 1993b), six risk factors were identified: smoking, diet and nutrition, obesity, blood pressure and alcohol.

CHD is often thought of as a disease of affluence – the result of rich diets, excessive alcohol and executive stress. In fact CHD, in common with most major causes of premature mortality, is more prevalent in manual than professional social groups. Despite the falling overall rate from coronary heart disease, numerous studies have demonstrated that the decline is more marked in higher socio-economic groups (Marmot and Dowel, 1986; Marmot et al., 1987; DoH, 1995b). CHD is typically viewed as a "male disease" and while mortality rates from CHD are considerably higher amongst men than they are amongst women, CHD remains the single greatest cause of death amongst women (Sharp, 1994; DoH, 1995a).

There are considerable variations in mortality from CHD among minority ethnic groups. Those born in the Indian subcontinent and East Africa have particularly high rates of CHD. A study of ethnic differences in death rates in England and Wales found that in 1988–92 mortality from CHD was 38% higher in men and 43% higher in women aged 20–69 who had been born in the Indian subcontinent than the rates for England and Wales as a whole (Balarajan, 1996). This differential rate in mortality cannot be fully accounted for by differences in diet, blood pressure and cigarette consumption. Various explanations have been put forward including the experience of stress exacerbated by the effects of racism (Francome and Marks, 1996). In addition, diabetes is more common amongst people from the Indian subcontinent, and this is linked to coronary heart disease. African-Caribbeans have lower than average levels of CHD, but hypertension is common as are high levels of stroke (almost twice as high as the average for England and Wales) (DoH, 1995b:86).

E xample

The Whitehall study of male civil servants compared CHD rates and risk factors among different employment grades. It found that lower grades had three times the CHD mortality of men in higher grades. Over 50% of the differences in CHD mortality rates could not be accounted for by standard risk factors including smoking, high blood pressure, blood cholesterol, lack of physical activity and being overweight. Employment grade was therefore a stronger predictor of risk than behaviour (Marmot *et al.*, 1978).

What factors associated with employment grade might be associated with the development of CHD?

Prevention of cardiovascular disease

Three levels of intervention to prevent CHD and stroke are typically promoted:

1. Primary prevention – preventing the onset of CHD and stroke in asymptomatic people.
2. Secondary prevention – preventing the progression of CHD and stroke in symptomatic people, by identifying and reducing risk behaviours.
3. Tertiary prevention – preventing avoidable complications of CHD and stroke and related conditions in those with established disease.

The "Health of the Nation" defined health promotion interventions narrowly as:

> "encourage and support individuals and communities to help themselves to improve health and prevent illness by changing to healthier lifestyles"

(DoH, 1993b:33).

Whilst there is some recognition of the wide range of agencies other than the NHS that need to be involved, and of the varied roles that different agencies can play, all of the interventions identified were underpinned by an individual behaviour change model of health promotion. There was an implicit assumption that lifestyle changes alone would bring about a reduction in ill-health and death from CHD and stroke. In a context where CHD and stroke are not thoroughly understood serious doubts have been raised about the applicability of individual behavioural interventions in the prevention of CHD (Oliver, 1992).

It has long been recognized that primary prevention programmes can be developed in two ways: by using a whole population approach or through selective targeting of individuals deemed to be at higher risk. The evidence from two large-scale studies, involving around 18,000 people, has been that preventive checks and advice from practice nurses in general practice is of little benefit (Family Heart Study Group, 1994; Muir *et al.*, 1994). The British Family Heart Study (Family Heart Study Group, 1994) concluded that individual screening and lifestyle advice did not achieve a significant reduction in cholesterol levels or behavioural changes. It concluded that targeting those with existing heart disease or known risk factors might be more beneficial. The OXCHECK study (a randomized controlled trial to assess the effectiveness of health checks by nurses in reducing risk factors for cardiovascular disease in patients aged 35–64) found that whilst there was no significant difference in smoking prevalence, quit rates or body mass index (BMI), systolic and diastolic blood pressure were 2.5% and 2.4% lower in the intervention group. The study concluded that although general health checks by nurses are ineffective in helping smokers to stop smoking they do help patients to modify their diet and total cholesterol level (Muir *et al.*, 1994). A systematic review of the role of health promotion in reducing the risk of CHD and stroke in older people over 55 years concluded that health promotion activities such as smoking advice and promoting physical activity needed to be targeted to those at higher risk of CHD and stroke (HEA, 1996a). The following findings were reported (Table 10.1).

D

The findings in Table 10.1 illustrate some of the difficulties in taking a risk factor approach to the prevention of coronary heart disease. How would you use these findings to develop a programme to reduce CHD? Using the evidence outlined above, what are the main difficulties in taking a risk factor approach to the prevention of CHD? What are the main implications for health promotion?

Table 10.1 *Health promotion interventions to reduce coronary heart disease and stroke amongst older people*

Reducing blood pressure

There is strong evidence to support medical treatment of (even mild) hypertension in younger and older people up to the age of 80–85.

Losing weight through exercise and taking fish oil supplements lower blood pressure in those with hypertension, but have little or no effect on those with normal blood pressure.

Relaxation methods have no demonstrable effect in lowering blood pressure.

Cutting down on salt seems to have a beneficial effect on people with high blood pressure.

Reducing alcohol intake can help reduce blood pressure in those with both high and normal blood pressure.

Lowering cholesterol

Using drugs to lower cholesterol may reduce deaths from CHD or the risk of it, but patients at low risk of CHD are unlikely to benefit much from treatment.

Reducing serum cholesterol through dietary changes can reduce cholesterol levels but has produced relatively small reductions in clinical trials.

Exercise on its own appears to have no long-term impact on cholesterol levels.

Multiple interventions

Interventions consisting of both drug and non-drug therapies were ineffective in reducing deaths from CHD and stroke, when used in the general population or workforces with a mean age of 50 years. However, there were reductions in studies which included those with high blood pressure.

Multiple risk factor intervention trials can modify risk factors, but the changes are relatively small.

Multiple risk factor intervention with or without exercise after a heart attack appears to be highly effective in reducing mortality.

Adapted from HEA, 1996a, with permission

There is a substantial amount of research that links nutrition and physical activity levels with CHD (e.g. HEA, 1993, 1995a, 1995b, 1996a, 1996b) and government action to date has focused on these two risk factors in addition to smoking, which is considered in Chapter 11.

Nutrition and healthy eating

Since the first Committee on the Medical Aspects of Food in 1984, the focus of government interventions on nutrition has been dietary recommendations. The 1994 COMA report recommended specific food consumption – for example, people should eat at least two portions of fish per week. However the strategies to help people to make these changes have centred on consumer education and advice, with little visible attempt to influence food production and sales (Calnan,

1991). Poor diet is attributed to inefficient food purchasing and budgeting, a preference for unhealthy food and a lack of knowledge concerning the value and composition of a healthy diet. Thus health promotion addresses these issues by advice on healthy eating or healthier cooking methods.

Yet many studies have shown that levels of knowledge about the constituents of a healthy diet are high and most people would prefer to eat a healthy diet (Lang *et al.*, 1984; Whitehead, 1988). As Figure 10.1 illustrates, purchasing and consumption patterns are influenced as much by national policies (including employment and benefit levels) and by the actions of distributors and retailers as by individual preference.

Substantial evidence shows how poverty affects food choice. A survey in 1994 by the National Children's Home suggested that 1.5 million families cannot afford to give their children a diet which was provided in an 1876 workhouse and that one in ten children regularly go without a meal (NCH, 1994). The 1993 National Food Survey (MAFF, 1994) showed that low income households are characterized by less dietary variety. Those shopping on a low income are unable to take advantage of low-cost supermarkets with their wide range of

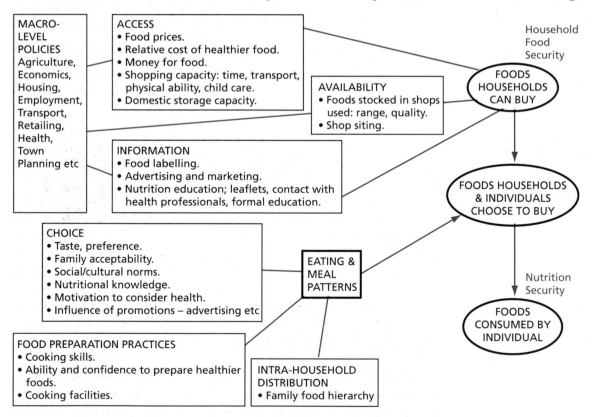

Figure 10.1   *Determinants of food and nutrition consumption (source: DoH Nutrition Task Force, 1996b, p. 4).*

produce and are restricted to local corner shops and mobile shops which are more expensive than other outlets (HEA, 1989). The unemployed, those on benefit payments or very low incomes, have the greatest difficulties and the worst diets (Dowler and Calvert, 1995). The priority is to have food which is calorie-rich and filling rather than that which is nutritious.

The Nutrition Task Force (Department of Health, 1996a) has identified four main priorities:

1. **The provision of education and information for the public** – e.g. "Balance of Good Health" was launched to professionals and health promoters in July 1994 by the Department of Health/MAFF/HEA and guidelines on educational materials have been produced.
2. **Catering providers are encouraged to provide more healthy food** – e.g. voluntary nutritional guidelines for hospital catering were launched in September 1995 and voluntary nutritional guidelines for those involved in the provision of school food are being produced.
3. **Influencing providers in the food chain** – e.g. working with industry to encourage them to reduce the fat content of foods and working with key players to consider the promotion of starchy foods, fish, fruit and vegetables.
4. **Working with NHS professionals** – e.g. a handbook for NHS managers was launched in June 1994 and a core nutrition curriculum document on the education of health professionals was launched in November 1994.

D How far do the actions in the above list address the factors influencing food choice which are illustrated in Figure 10.1?

C ase study

St Pancras Day Centre

Between 1980 and 1992 the number of food retail outlets decreased by 35% from 121,600 to 78,606, at the expense of small retailers (DoH, 1996b:6). The number of large retail outlets (particularly in town centres) has also decreased in favour of the development of superstores located on the edge of town centres. The concentration of food retailing makes access to low cost, healthy foods including fresh fruit and vegetables particularly difficult for those on a low income, those dependent on public transport and in rural areas. There are numerous local projects which aim to improve the availability of and access to healthier food including cookery skills courses, community cafes and lunch clubs and food co-operatives (HEA/National Food Alliance, 1997). Other projects have attempted to minimize the impact of fewer retail outlets.

The St Pancras Day Centre, as part of its services for older people, established a small food shop in 1994. It was started with a small grant during the European Year of the Elderly. The grant paid for initial start-up costs; shelving and stock for the shop. The shop provides basic affordable groceries for older people such as sugar, toilet rolls, small

The Balance of Good Health

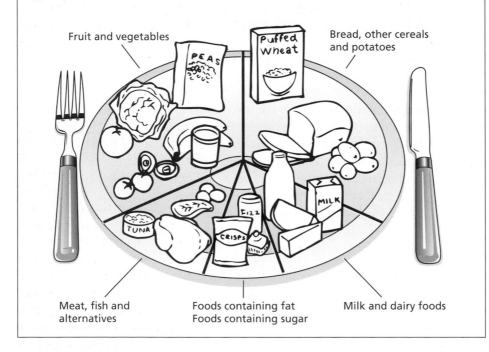

Fruit and vegetables

Bread, other cereals and potatoes

Meat, fish and alternatives

Foods containing fat
Foods containing sugar

Milk and dairy foods

Figure 10.2 *Balance of good health (adapted from a poster in HEA, 1996, with permission).*

sizes of storable items, rather than items which are usually considered healthier like dried pulses and vegetables. The shop makes no direct attempt to encourage healthier options but seeks primarily to address the difficulties of low income shopping. The shop enables housebound people, who visit the centre for other activities, to buy items whilst they are there. They would not normally be able to shop for themselves and this service affords this client group some independence. The staff have kept the shop to a small scale, opening once a week, and on demand to regular users. The shop pays for itself but makes no profit – money from sales is used to replenish stocks, which is done from cash and carry sources. The food shop is an important part of the services offered and runs alongside a luncheon club, social activities and a range of advice and information to older people. It is an example of a local service, which though small, adds to vulnerable older people's quality of life and independence.

Should projects which address nutrition in low income groups always seek to promote healthier options?

Action to tackle the food problems of deprived communities cannot be done, according to the Department of Health's Low Income Task Force, outside mainstream food retailing (DoH, 1996b:19). As part of a Health Plan for Camden as a Healthy City, an audit of food retailers is being undertaken. This will form the starting point for a local food partnership between statutory agencies and retailers to tackle the problems of poverty and food.

Physical activity

Over the last 25 years mounting evidence has pointed to the benefits of regular physical activity in protecting against osteoporosis, in reducing blood pressure and in improving a sense of well-being (Fentem *et al.*, 1988). Yet evidence from the Allied Dunbar National Fitness Survey in 1990 found that current levels of activity in the UK are low and that 70% do not take enough exercise at work or in their leisure time to benefit their health (Sports Council/HEA, 1992). Twenty nine per cent of men and 28% of women can be categorized as sedentary and 30% of men and 50% of women aged 65–74 have insufficient strength in their muscles to rise from a chair without using their arms. The majority of the sample believed however, that they were very or fairly fit. Public perceptions of physical activity were that it is associated with sport and therefore is something for which time needs to be made available and for which special clothes need to be bought.

The Physical Activity Task Force was established in 1993 to develop a national strategy to promote physical activity. The consultation paper "More people, more active, more often" (DoH, 1995a) recognizes that moderate activity should be the focus of a national strategy as this is a more realistic goal for the population. The Health Education Authority correspondingly launched a three year campaign in 1996 called "Active for Life" which seeks to raise awareness of the benefits of 30 minutes moderate physical activity on most days of the week.

A review of the effectiveness of physical activity intervention studies among the general public (Hillsdon *et al.*, 1995) found that those interventions that were effective in attracting and sustaining high levels of participation had the following features in common:

- home-based activity, rather than structured programmes based in a special facility or centre;
- informal and unsupervised exercise;
- frequent professional contact for encouragement, either by telephone or home visit;
- moderate intensity exercise;
- the activity is enjoyable and convenient and can be completed in three sessions per week.

Accordingly, Hillsdon *et al.* (1995) see walking as satisfying all of these criteria.

The focus of most work on physical activity has been on the individual making behavioural changes, yet the barriers facing different population groups vary considerably. Asian women surveyed in Bristol for example, cited the following as barriers to increasing their activity levels (Pilgrim *et al.*, 1993):

- burden of other duties;
- fear of racism (including when out walking);
- language difficulties;
- inappropriateness of facilities including dress code, male/female provision, high cost.

As Taylor (1996) puts it:

> "access to equipment, programmes and safe places to be active is determined to a great extent by socio-economic status."

Unless specific groups are targeted, most schemes have inadvertently attracted middle aged, middle class women. The greatest potential for health gain would be achieved by targeting to ensure that leisure-based schemes are more appropriate for and accessible to low socio-economic groups, unemployed men (especially those who are also from low socio-economic groups), and older people.

The Physical Activity Task Force identified children as a specific group to be targeted to increase their levels of activity. Changing social trends such as increased television viewing and concerns about personal safety have led to a reduction in cycling and walking as the mainstay of children's activity. In 1971, for example, most nine year olds walked to school on their own. In 1990 only 50% would make that journey on foot if it entailed crossing a road (Hillman *et al.*, 1990, 1993). Fear of road traffic accidents means that the majority of primary school children are driven to school. The introduction of the National Curriculum in schools, together with the reduction in teachers' involvement in extracurricular activity, has led to a reduction in PE lessons and sport. Behavioural patterns established in childhood do exert an influence on later adult behaviour and cardiovascular risk factors can be found even in childhood, hence the concern to encourage children to build physical activity into their lives (WHO, 1990).

The association between activity and sport is also evident in GP referral to exercise schemes at leisure centres. Yet a review of physical activity promotion in primary care settings (Biddle *et al.*, 1994) found that there was little, if any, good quality evaluation of whether such schemes are effective in encouraging a sustained increase in physical activity. Exercise schemes which "prescribe" subsidized exercise at leisure centres, although popular, have failed to recruit sufficient numbers of people and/or to make an impact on people's levels of physical activity (Iliffe *et al.*, 1994; Taylor, 1996). The randomized controlled trial carried out in Hailsham found no discernible difference in levels of physical activity between the intervention group and the control group at 37 weeks. Attending a leisure centre does not seem to be the most effective way to increase levels of physical activity for many people. Indications from trials currently underway in the UK and USA suggest, however, that targeted promotion of physical activity to individuals with conditions for whom exercise is known to be particularly beneficial (for example, non-insulin dependent diabetes, myocardial infarction, depression, hypertension) is likely to be effective in the primary care setting (Hillsdon, personal communication).

Research has suggested that schemes which increase participation can have long-term gain. The workplace is a setting where benefits for workforce participants compared with non-participants have been shown. However, typical participation rates in exercise schemes have been shown to be low (20–40% of eligible employees) and drop out rates tend to be high.

Case study

Health at Work in the NHS

In 1992 the Health Education Authority set up the Health at Work in the NHS initiative to support the government's "Health of the Nation" strategy. Its aim was to improve the health of NHS staff by introducing healthy workplace programmes in NHS premises. It is suggested that the NHS as a major employer (5% total workforce) should act as an exemplar by providing an environment for staff that offers opportunities for the adoption of positive health practices.

The Health at Work initiative includes a quality standard for physical activity which identifies what NHS premises need to achieve:

- a comprehensive physical activity policy;
- raise awareness and motivate staff to be more active, e.g. instituting a stair climbing week;
- provide fit breaks, worksite trim trails and publish routes for lunchtime walks;
- offer on-site classes, e.g. Look After Yourself, yoga;
- liaise with local leisure centres to offer discounts;

■   provide changing rooms, showers and safe bike racks.

Studies from America have shown, however, that such schemes have low recruitment (Dishman, 1988) and those who do attend are those already active and participating in fitness schemes outside work.

> **R** Which of the following would you regard as the most important factors in encouraging participation in a workplace activity programme?
> ■ an incentive or reward;
> ■ longer lunch breaks;
> ■ identification of employee needs;
> ■ graded classes to accommodate varying abilities;
> ■ proximity of any programme;
> ■ small groups;
> ■ support from senior management;
> ■ opportunity for partners and families to be involved.

The Health at Work in the NHS initiative arises from the World Health Organization view that health needs to be promoted in the settings in which people live and work and that such settings not only provide an ideal opportunity for health education but also affect people's health in their organizational systems. Issues such as communication and power structures, resource distribution and the autonomy of employees are all significant factors. Whilst health might be seen as a natural priority of the NHS, its corporate culture and work pressures militate against this. The biggest obstacle to workplace health promotion is thus a culture of task achievement.

Some workplace programmes have the potential to stimulate more active living by developing policies and incentives to encourage use of public transport and/or walking and cycling to get to work. Camden & Islington Health Authority reviewed the potential NHS contribution and identified a number of relevant areas including:

■   incentives to use public transport, cycling or walking as a means of transport to work;
■   limited car parking and low mileage rates to deter the use of private cars for work journeys;
■   efficient use of cars through vehicle fleets and incentives to encourage car sharing (Lewis, 1996).

Southampton University Hospital Trust have introduced a £50 incentive to encourage staff to swap their cars for alternative forms of transport. If bicycles are used for business journeys a mileage rate above that for cars is offered (Moore, 1995). Staff living within a mile of the trust are unable to park in hospital car parks except in special circumstances such as mobility difficulties. Since the introduction of the scheme cycling among staff has increased by 70% (Owen and Davis, 1995).

> **R**
>
> To what extent are your own levels of physical activity dependent on transport policies and employment practices? Taking your workplace and your community as an example, how would you respond to the following comments?
> ■ "If I cycle to the shops will there be anywhere to chain my bike?"
> ■ "Is it safe to let my child walk to school?"
> ■ "If I cycle to work is there anywhere to get changed?"
> ■ "If I go out for a run at lunchtime will people think I'm skiving off work?"

C ase study

Camden transport policy

Developing transport policy at a local level is a complex task requiring major intersectoral collaboration and commitment at all levels. Government policy on transport and land use sets out as one of its prime objectives the reduction of growth in the length and number of motorized journeys and general reduction on the reliance on private vehicles (DoE and DoT, 1994). Local authorities are committed to reducing traffic growth and reliance upon cars in central London. This is generally approached through planning and engineering routes within local authorities and, more recently, through Local Agenda 21 (which arose out of the global plan for sustainable development produced at the Rio Earth Summit in 1992). At the same time, choices which are made about transport options are generally seen as private choices. Improving transport in order to protect health is not yet fully established as a legitimate health objective. Indeed the proposed targets for the Health of the Nation Environment key area (DoH, 1997a) did not even acknowledge the health implications of transport policy. However, immediately after its election the new Labour government made a commitment to reducing private car transport in order to protect the environment. The Environment Minister speaking at a conference to launch the new health strategy "Our Healthier Nation" announced proposals for "a transport system that is efficient, clean, safe and that provides genuine choice. It must respect the environment, and take account of the costs that transport itself imposes. More pedestrians and cyclists would mean not only fewer cars on the roads, but also that we could become a fitter and more active generation" (DoH, 1997b:9).

While there are opportunities for common objectives on specific initiatives the role of public health and (by extension) health authorities, is not always clear to those working in areas traditionally perceived to hold expertise on transport issues. In Camden and Islington, as in many other areas, developing joint work on transport policy is a useful "test case" of some of the difficulties in trying to achieve health as a higher priority across all sectors (Jones, 1993). In Camden and Islington the Health Authority recognize that transport policies and choices have a significant impact on health. The Director of Public Health has been instrumental in raising the profile of the wider health implications of transport policy; in particular, in promoting the development of a more health-oriented transport system (which has as its priorities: access and provision for all social groups; a reduction in the use of private vehicles; an increase in cycling and walking; promotion of increased physical activity). These goals have been differentially taken on in each of the two London Boroughs. In Islington these goals have been prioritized by the Director of Environment and Technical Services and are in line with his vision of the council's role in achieving national road safety targets, local implementation of Local Agenda

21, targets set by the Department of the Environment and local political support. The role of public health is seen as one which complements and enhances the local authority's responsibilities. Conversely, in Camden, whilst there is considerable joint work in developing and commissioning an integrated community transport system, there is less focus on the wider health implications. The Environment Directorate see this area of work as one in which they have the expertise and perceive the more traditional planning, traffic management and engineering roles to be the priorities. This is not surprising when there are major trunk roads and red routes dividing the borough. Consequently, the involvement of public health and the public health agenda is seen as duplicating work that is already ongoing or as creating new work which is not a current priority. Whilst there is agreement that the development of a more health-oriented transport policy is important the different agendas of the agencies involved make progress in this area difficult to achieve (Jones, 1993:42).

D Transport policies impact on health in many different ways. What are the implications of transport policies for
- physical activity levels
- pollution
- accidents
- social mobility and isolation?

What barriers are there to integrating health concerns in transport policies? How might these barriers be addressed?

The case study on transport policy shows clearly how the agendas of health and sustainable development are inextricably linked. For example, a planning policy which encourages the revival of town centres and the growth of self-contained communities will impact on health by reducing the need to travel short distances by car and make cycling and walking more feasible. Policies to reduce the use of motor vehicles (e.g. pedestrianization schemes in town centres, road pricing, improvements in public transport, cheaper freight rail transport) encourage other modes of transport which promote physical activity (Hillman, 1991).

Conclusion

Cardiovascular disease is a condition for which there are known risk factors. Most CHD and stroke prevention work has concentrated on reducing these risk factors, which are often viewed as separate elements of an individual's lifestyle. A greater understanding of the factors affecting, and often constraining, people's lifestyle choices, has led to a more sophisticated awareness of the complexity of changing behaviour. The case studies in this chapter illustrate how inter-agency working, and collaboration on policy formation and implementation can have profound effects on people's behaviour.

These case studies are examples of how the traditional approach to lifestyle change can be broadened to include wider aspects of health. Broader activities, such as an integrated transport policy, will have several positive effects in increasing physical activity levels, reducing air and noise pollution, and lowering the accident rate. This chapter has shown how work undertaken within a traditional medical model of risk factor reduction and prevention can be enhanced by the application of health promotion principles of equity, collaboration and participation.

Further discussion

■ How appropriate is it to address individual risk factors for cardiovascular disease?

■ What problems are there with including core health promotion principles in cardiovascular prevention programmes?

Recommended reading

■ Department of Health (1993) *Key area Handbook, Coronary Heart Disease and Stroke*, London, HMSO.
Department of Health (1995) *More People, More Active, More Often*, London, HMSO.
Department of Health (1996) *Low income, food, nutrition and health: strategies for Improvement*, London, HMSO.
The Department of Health have issued these reports which outline the priorities for achieving a reduction in cardiovascular disease and how to plan interventions.

■ Draper P (1991) (ed.) *Health through Public Policy*, London, Green Print.
A useful book which illustrates the overlapping policy areas of the environment and public health.

■ HEA (1993) *Health Update 1: Coronary Heart Disease*, London, Health Education Authority.
HEA (1995) *Health Update no. 5: Physical Activity*, London, Health Education Authority.
The above booklets from the Health Education Authority provide brief summaries of the epidemiology of these risk factors and examples of health promotion interventions.

■ Holmes R (1993) "Coronary heart disease: a cautionary tale", in Davey B and Popay J (eds) *Dilemmas in Health Care*, Buckingham, Open University Press.
Examines the arguments for CHD prevention in the face of uncertainty about its causes.

■ Rose G (1992) *The strategy of Preventive Medicine*, Oxford, Oxford University Press.
An interesting and accessible discussion of prevention strategies based on risk factor identification and population-based strategies.

References

Balarajan R (1996) "Ethnicity and variation in mortality from coronary heart disease", *Health Trends*, **28**(2), 45–51.

Biddle S *et al.* (1994) *Physical Activity Promotion in Primary Health Care in England*, London, Health Education Authority.

Calnan M (1991) *Preventing Coronary Heart Disease: Prospects, Policies and Politics*, London, Routledge.

Department of the Environment & Department of Transport (1994) *Planning Policy Guidance: Transport*, London, HMSO.

Department of Health (1992) *The Health of the Nation: A Strategy for Health in England*, London, HMSO.

Department of Health (1993a) *Health Survey for England*, London, HMSO.

Department of Health (1993b) *Key area Handbook, Coronary Heart Disease & Stroke*, London, HMSO.

Department of Health (1995a) *More People, More Active, More Often*, London, HMSO.

Department of Health (1995b) *Variations in Health: What can the Department of Health and the NHS do?* London, HMSO.

Department of Health (1996a) *Eat Well II: A progress report from the Nutrition Task Force on the action plan to achieve the Health of the Nation targets on diet and nutrition*, London, Department of Health.

Department of Health Nutrition Task Force (1996b) *Low Income, Food, Nutrition and Health: Strategies for Improvement*, London, HMSO.

Department of Health (1997a) *The Health of the Nation on Environmental Health*, London, HMSO.

Department of Health (1997b) *Target: Our Healthier Nation*, London, Department of Health.

Dishman (1988) *Exercise adherence and its impact on public health*, Champaign, Illinois, Human Kinetics Books.

Dowler E and Calvert C (1995) *Nutrition and diet in lone-parent families in London*, London, Family Policy Studies Centre.

Family Heart Study Group (1994) "Randomised controlled trials evaluating cardiovascular screening and intervention in general practice: principal results of the British Family Heart Study", *British Medical Journal*, **308**, 313–20.

Fentem PH, Bassey RJ, Turnbull MB (1988) *The new case for exercise*, London, Sports Council/Health Education Authority.

Francome C and Marks DF (1996) *Improving the Health of the Nation: The failure of the government's health reforms*, London, Middlesex University Press.

HEA (1989) *Diet, Nutrition and Healthy Eating in Low Income Groups*, London, Health Education Authority.

HEA (1993) *Health Update 1: Coronary Heart Disease*, London, Health Education Authority.

HEA (1995a) *Health Update no. 5: Physical Activity*, London, Health Education Authority.

HEA (1995b) *Promoting physical activity: guidance for commissioners, purchasers and providers*, London, Health Education Authority.

HEA (1996a) *Health promotion in older people for the prevention of coronary heart disease and stroke*, London, Health Education Authority.

HEA (1996b) *Nutritional aspects of cardiovascular disease*, London, Health Education Authority.

HEA/National Food Alliance (1997) *Food and Low Income Database*, London, Health Education Authority.

Hillman M (1991) "Health transport policy", in Draper P (ed.) *Health Through Public Policy*, London, Green Print.

Hillman M, Adams J and Whittled J (1990) *One false move: a study of children's independent mobility*, London, Policy Studies Institute.

Hillman M, Adams J and Whittled J (1993) *Children, transport and quality of life*, London, Policy Studies Institute.

Hillsdon, M, Thorogood M, Antis T and Morris J N (1995) "Randomised controlled trials of physical activity promotion in free-living populations: a review", *Journal of Epidemiology and Community Health*, **49**, 448–53.

Illiffe S, Tai Gould M, Thorogood M, Hillsdon M (1994) "Prescribing exercise in general practice", *British Medical Journal*, **309**:494-95.

Jones L (1993) *Health and Wellbeing workbook 3 Health on Wider Agendas*, Milton Keynes, Open University Press.

Lang T, Andrews H, Bedale C and Hannon E (1984) *Jam tomorrow*, Manchester, Food Policy Unit, Manchester Polytechnic.

Le Fanu J (1991) "A healthy diet–fact or fashion?", in Berber P, Kristen I, Mills M *et al.*, *Health, Lifestyle and Environment*, London, the Social Affairs Unit/Manhattan Institute.

Lewis J (1996) *Transport, Environment and Health in the NHS in Camden and Islington*, London, Camden & Islington Public Health Department.

MAFF (1994) *Household food consumption and expenditure*, London, HMSO.

Marmot M G and Dowel M E (1986) "Mortality decline and widening social inequalities", *Lancet*, **1**, 274–276.

Marmot M G, Rose G and Shipley M (1978) "Employment grade and coronary heart disease in British civil servants", *Journal of Epidemiology and Community Health*, **32**, 244–49.

Marmot M G, Shipley M G and Rose G (1987) "Inequalities in death-specific explanations of a general pattern?" *Lancet*, **1**, 1104.

Moore W (1995) "On your bike", *Healthlines*, **23**, 20–21.

Muir J, Mant D, Jones L and Yudkin P (1994) "Effectiveness of health checks conducted by nurses in primary care: results of the OXCHECK study after one year", *British Medical Journal*, January 29, 308–12.

NCH (1994) *Poverty and Nutrition Survey*, London, National Children's Home.

Oliver M (1992) "Doubts about preventing coronary heart disease", *British Medical Journal*, **304**, 393–94.

Owen L and Davis A (1995) "Life Cycle", *Health Service Journal*, 24 August.

Pilgrim S with Fenton S, Hughes T, Hine C and Tibbs N (1993) *The Bristol Black and Ethnic Minorities Health Survey*, Bristol, University of Bristol.

Sharp I (ed) (1994) *CHD: Are Women Special?*, London, National Forum for CHD Prevention.

Sports Council/HEA (1992) *Allied Dunbar National Fitness Survey*, London, Sports Council/Health Education Authority.

Taylor A (1996) *Evaluating GP exercise referral schemes: findings from a randomised control study*, London, Chelsea School Research Centre, Topic Report No 6.

Whitehead M (1988) *The Health Divide*, London, Penguin.

WHO (1990) *Prevention in childhood and youth of adult cardiovascular disease: time for action*, Geneva: World Health Organization.

11 *Cancer prevention*

Jennie Naidoo, Vicki Taylor and Jane Wills

Key points

- National health strategy and lung, skin, breast and cervical cancers.
- Evidence of effective interventions.
- Screening programmes.
- Smoking reduction.

Overview

Cancers are a major cause of death and ill health, accounting for about 25% of all deaths in 1991 (DoH, 1992). Some cancers can now be prevented by risk factor reduction, or cured following early detection through screening and self-examination. This chapter reviews the evidence of effective interventions to prevent four cancers – lung, skin, breast and cervical cancers. It focuses in detail on the range of health promotion strategies to prevent and reduce smoking, the major risk factor for lung cancer. It also looks at the national screening programmes for breast and cervical cancers and ways in which inequities in health status can be reduced by making the screening service more accessible and acceptable.

Introduction

The following statistics about cancer are notable (Thames Cancer Registry, 1995):

- Over 300,000 people develop cancer in the UK each year and over half that number die from it.
- Cancer accounts for one in four deaths in England.
- One in three people will develop cancer before they are 75.
- More than 70% of cancers are diagnosed in people aged 60 and over.
- More than half the deaths in women aged 35–55 are due to cancer.

Four cancers were identified in the "Health of the Nation" strategy: lung, skin, breast and cervical. Although other cancers (e.g. prostate, colon) contribute significantly to mortality and morbidity rates, the cancers chosen have the greatest potential for improvements in health and quality of life through screening, diagnosis, treatment and rehabilitation. Evidence of effective health promotion and disease prevention interventions existed (especially for lung cancer) and these provided significant scope for adding years to life. Finally, it was possible to set specific outcome targets and to monitor progress towards them (DoH, 1992).

It is often thought that the increase in incidence of cancers is a product of the extended lifespans achieved as a result of the decline in infectious diseases. This is only partly true. Whilst the incidence of cancers rises with age, most are associated with poverty, disadvantage and deprivation (e.g. the incidence of lung and cervical cancer is greatest in lower social classes). There is also information from epidemiological and clinical studies linking risk factors to certain types of cancer. For example, it is well known that smoking is related to various cancers, especially lung cancer, and that exposure to ultraviolet radiation is linked to skin cancer.

Cancer, despite being dreaded, is now also seen as a preventable disease in many cases. Health promotion has focused on primary prevention (health education and support for behaviour changes) and secondary prevention (early detection and treatment of pre-cancerous cell changes). However, primary prevention aims to influence the known risk factors for cancer through information and support for behaviour change, and through selective screening programmes. Environmental pollution, exposure to toxic materials and changes in the quality of food have all been linked to cancer. Yet there has been very little cancer prevention activity focused on environments or healthy public policies (with the exception of support for smoke-free environments).

Lung cancer

Lung cancer accounts for 25% of all cancer deaths in England. Primary lung cancer is the most frequently occurring tumour in men and the third most frequent in women (DoH, 1993) although it is rare in those aged under 35. It has been estimated that up to 90% of the causes of lung cancers are associated with active or passive smoking (Greenwald and Sondick, 1986) and smoking is also associated with an increased risk of other cancers (e.g. mouth, oesophagus, throat). It appears that the longer an individual is exposed to tobacco smoke, the higher the risk of developing the disease (Doll, 1990). Other factors, such as occupational exposure to asbestos or other minerals, and environmental factors such as radon gas, can interact with smoking to cause lung cancer. Lung cancer is therefore most common in those socio-economic and population groups whose exposure to tobacco smoke and occupational risk factors is greatest (OPCS, 1992). There is a clear association between deprivation and smoking – not only are poorer groups more likely to become smokers but having become smokers they are also least likely to give up (Marsh and McKay, 1994). One striking figure is the high number of lone parents who smoke (nearly 70%) (Figures 11.1a and b).

Figure 11.1 *Changes in smoking prevalence in men (a) and women (b), 1976–1990, by income quarter and family type among respondents aged 16–44 (from Marsh and Mackay, 1994). Key: ---- lone parents; —— married, with children; ..... married, no children; ---not married, no children.*

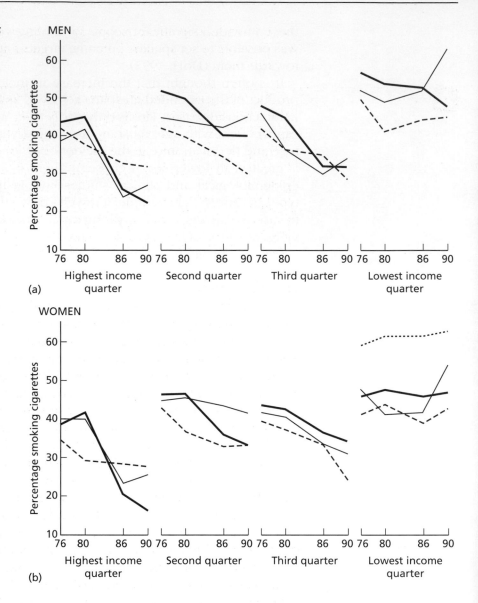

Approaches to smoking prevention

By far the greatest scope for reducing ill-health and death from lung cancer is through smoking prevention and cessation. Smoking is the most important cause of avoidable ill-health and premature death in England and the health problems associated with smoking are now known to be considerably greater than in the original report by the Royal College of Physicians (RCP, 1962). The Cancers Key Area Handbook (DoH, 1993:30) identified five approaches to prevention:

1. Health education on the effects of smoking.
2. Action to stop people from starting to smoke.
3. Helping people to stop.

D Smoking has become increasingly concentrated among poor people, especially among poor women. What are the implications of this for health promotion?

4. Protecting non-smokers from passive smoking.
5. Preventing occupational exposures causally associated with lung cancer.

Activity

In the table below identify interventions which are examples of the different approaches to smoking prevention.

Aim	Intervention
Health education	
Prevention	
Cessation	
Protection	

Health education

Most of the research on the impact of smoking on health has focused on the relationship between the behaviour and the disease. Most strategies to reduce smoking behaviour are based on the assumption that somehow smokers do not know that smoking is harmful and therefore need more information. Mass media campaigns, advice from health practitioners and education in schools have all stressed the risks to health from smoking. Yet 70% smokers want to give up and are well aware of its risks (OPCS, 1994). Theories of behaviour change, as we saw in Chapter 2, dominate in the field of health promotion and one explanation for the apparently irrational decision of smokers to continue smoking is a lack of motivation. One of the most accepted health promotion strategies is to increase smokers' motivation to quit by the advice and support of a respected professional – the general practitioner. Early studies showed that after receiving opportunistic advice from a GP within a routine consultation, six out of ten smokers may try to stop and 5% of these may succeed (Russell *et al.*, 1979). A meta-analysis (see Chapter 3 for an explanation of methods of reviewing effectiveness) of 39 controlled trials of various GP interventions concluded that 5.8% of smokers stopped for 12 months, and that GP advice gave the best and most consistent results in smoking cessation (Reid *et al.*, 1992). Other members of the primary care team also have a role in smoking cessation. Table 11.1 below summarizes some of the evidence relating to the effectiveness, showing that advice as well as information significantly increases cessation rates.

Smoking needs to be placed in a wider context than merely as a lifestyle choice. The high smoking rates of those under stress from unemployment, poverty, isolation and caring responsibilities suggest that smoking serves to reduce stress (Graham, 1993; Marsh and McKay, 1994). Whether this is through a direct effect on mood or whether smokers continue smoking to avoid the stress of withdrawal

Table 11.1 *Smoking prevention activities of health professionals*

Practice nurses	A small but significant additional effect of nurse advice following GP referral – 3.3% reduction in smoking prevalence with GP advice alone to 4.7% reduction using nurse advice – useful support role for those motivated to stop smoking (Sanders, 1992). The OXCHECK study suggests that smoking cessation advice offered to smokers within a general health promotion programme, was ineffective (ICRF, 1994). The British Family Heart Study had disappointing results – reduction in smoking prevalence in the intervention groups was 1.0% for men and 0.7% for women (Family Heart Study Group, 1994).
Pharmacists	In an ideal position to reinforce health education messages. No research into effectiveness. Could consider interventions which combine client purchase of transdermal nicotine patches with pharmacist advice (Russell *et al.*, 1993).
Professions allied to medicine (PAMS)	No research evidence into effectiveness of PAMs. Could consider pilot interventions with, e.g. chiropodists, dentists or physiotherapists, in consultations where other relevant risk factors are present. Possibly combined with distribution of nicotine patches.
Health visitors and other community nurses	Little evidence available. Two trials incorporating advice from health visitors with that of doctors did not demonstrate significant additional effects, although other studies show them to be as effective as doctors. Community nurses can increase smoking cessation rates if trained in counselling skills, and one study demonstrated a 17% success rate after one year (Clark *et al.*, 1990).
Family planning doctors	A USA study demonstrated validated cessation rates of 3.7% with advice from a family planning physician compared with only 0.09% with information only (Li *et al.*, 1984).
Practice counsellors	On-going support can provide significant effects, especially if combined with self-help materials. Validated cessation rate at six months in one USA study showed a 6.3% rate compared with 1.2% for information only (Weissfeld and Holloway, 1991).

is much debated. Although GPs are recommended to use a protocol for managing smokers, this does not include the offer of nicotine replacement which is routinely prescribed in the USA.

The use of media campaigns, paid advertising and unpaid publicity

The precise contribution which media campaigns can play in encouraging smokers to quit remains disputed. One series of studies found that up to 5% of smokers quit long term after exposure to media campaigns, whilst others have found either no impact at all or differential impact with young people being most influenced by media advertising (Reid *et al.*, 1992; Townsend *et al.*, 1994). Paid advertising to promote smoking cessation is very expensive but it does lead to a great deal of unpaid coverage. The creation of unpaid publicity affects public opinion which in turn, encourages governments to introduce tighter controls through taxation and advertising restrictions (Chapman and Lupton, 1994). Reid (1996:340) thus concludes that the generation of unpaid publicity is probably the most cost-effective form of health education.

Activity

If you were writing a press release to promote non-smoking, which of the following aspects would you prioritize and why?

- Local angle – statistics, trends, services available.
- Local celebrities used as role models.
- Information – basic details about health risks.
- Positive message – stressing the benefits of smoking cessation.
- Support for non-smokers rights, e.g. to be free from passive smoking in public places.
- Targeted at young people and/or poor people.
- Sources of further information and support.

Education of young people

In England, an average of 10% of young people aged 12 to 13 smoke regularly (Lader and Matheson, 1991; HEA, 1992). Smoking among boys aged 14 has declined from 18% to 12% in the last ten years, smoking amongst girls aged 14 has gone up from 14% to 16% (Faculty of Public Health Medicine, 1993). There is little evidence for the effectiveness of either stopping smoking in teenagers or preventing them from smoking in the first place. The impact of smoking education programmes in schools has been well researched. Nutbeam *et al.* (1993) suggest health education programmes in schools have no discernible impact on established smoking behaviour. Reid *et al.* (1992) concluded that school programmes can delay the onset of smoking and may help some parents to stop. The evaluation of an early smoking prevention project found that boys taking part in the "My Body" programme were less likely to smoke at 11 than their matched controls, whilst girls taking part were more likely to smoke than a matched control group (Murray, 1982). For young people, smoking carries associations of maturity and rebellion which are attractive to some adolescents (HEA, 1992). Stead *et al.* (1996:34) thus conclude that the most successful programmes are those which

> "focus on raising awareness of the socio-cultural pressures to smoke and on developing skills to resist those pressures. Information on short-term effects of smoking should be included but information about long-term health risks is unlikely to have a significant effect, and programmes should use interactive learning methods such as role play and pupil led discussion".

There is also evidence that schools and colleges with a no smoking policy have fewer smokers and less smoking among students (Cancer Research Campaign, 1991).

D

Which of the following activities would you recommend to reduce teenage smoking and why?

- Curriculum lessons on smoking (in biology on the constituents of cigarettes and their effects on the body).
- Peer education programme using young people themselves to educate others about smoking and alcohol.
- Complete smoking ban in school.
- Theatre in Education play about smoking.
- Carbon monoxide testing of students.

D What practical and ethical problems can you see in extending the following current legislative measures to control smoking?

- Ban on sale of cigarettes to minors.
- Encouraging smoke-free environments.
- Discouraging smoking through taxation.
- Voluntary agreements on advertising and promotion.

Legislative action

Trying to prevent young people from starting to smoke is an accepted health promotion strategy. Yet as we saw in the previous section, education programmes have had limited success. Restricting access to and the supply of the product through the Children and Tobacco Act 1991 is therefore one way of trying to reduce smoking in young people. Yet the law is virtually impossible to police and cigarettes are easily accessible to young people. Almost 75% of young people under 16 who smoke regularly buy cigarettes from a shop once a week and 50% of retailers sell cigarettes to obviously underage children (Stead *et al.*, 1996).

Although there is a ban on smoking on public transport and, increasingly, other public places and workplaces are smoke-free, there is some reluctance by government to extend the legislation. Restricting smoking at work is principally to protect non-smokers from the environmental effects of tobacco and to protect employers from the possibility of litigation. Yet few ex-smokers cite workplace restrictions as a reason for quitting and there is little evidence that workplace policies in themselves reduce prevalence (Ben Shlomo *et al.*, 1991).

The relationship between the price of cigarettes and consumption is very close – a rise in price of 1% generally causes a decline in consumption by 0.5% (Townsend *et al.*, 1994). Reid *et al.* (1992:193) conclude that "fiscal policy has a much larger influence on consumption than any of the other interventions". However, the known link between poverty and smoking (Marsh and Mackay, 1994) means that tobacco taxation is a clear example of "regressive" taxation which impacts disproportionately on poorer people.

The new Labour government has committed itself to extending the previously voluntary controls on tobacco advertising. The Minister for Public Health is committed to banning tobacco advertising and phasing out sports sponsorship by tobacco companies. Other proposals to be considered include reducing nicotine levels in cigarettes, increasing the legal age at which cigarettes can be purchased from 16 to 18 years and listing the chemical contents of tobacco on cigarette packets.

D There is an explicit national strategy to address drug misuse (Home Office, 1994) but no similar strategy for tobacco use. Why do you think this is?

Case study

The use of drama

The evidence that smoking is more prevalent in particular population groups has led to the targeting of these groups on the assumption that such groups are "hard to reach" with conventional educational messages and that somehow the message is failing to get through.

A survey by East London and City Health Authority suggested that the prevalence of smoking is extremely high in Turkish communities (92% of Turkish men were found to be medium to heavy smokers). The survey also found the Turkish population to have a lower level of awareness of smoking-related diseases compared to the general population. A Turkish language drama has been developed in neighbouring Camden and Islington and is being performed in community centres and Turkish cafes.

It has become increasingly common to use drama as an educational tool which can "harness the techniques and imaginative potency of theatre" (Jackson, 1993:1). The experience of Theatre in Education projects with young people has been that drama readily engages and enables the audience to personalize issues on an emotional as well as a factual level (Power, 1995:29).

One of the important criteria for effective educational theatre is the credibility of the company and the degree to which the audience can empathize with the characters. "Tiyatro Ala-turka" theatre company were chosen for this work because they specialize in bilingual theatre and use materials from Anatolian theatrical sources, i.e. puppets, shadow plays and tuluat (improvization). Traditionally, Anatolian cultures have identified with puppetry more than live theatre. A Turkish script writer who had worked closely with the community was approached to discuss the aims of the drama. These were:

- to raise general awareness of smoking;
- to change the audience's perception of smoking;

■   to raise issues about passive smoking.

For drama education to be effective it needs to be created out of a knowledge of the group for whom it is being devised. Every aspect of this programme from the content of the play to the staging to the company members themselves was developed for its Turkish audience. After the script was completed it was evaluated by other Turkish speaking healthcare workers and amended. The project was intended to be interactive and it was expected that the audience would ask questions during the performance. The actors thus become facilitators and need to have credibility in their role as health educators. Prior to rehearsal the actors were given some training so that they had a better understanding of smoking-related issues. This consisted of

■   information on the smoking habits of the Turkish speaking community in London and in Turkey;
■   factors affecting health and the role of health promotion;
■   information on various smoking issues;
■   a brief introduction to the cycle of change involved in stopping smoking;
■   smoking as a risk factor in relation to other social issues such as unemployment, poor housing, immigration and poverty.

The play lasted ten minutes and the discussion took no more than twenty minutes. In addition to its ability to engage audiences, theatre is also a mobile form of communication. This play is therefore ideally suited for touring and can be performed within the context of other events such as political meetings or special celebrations. The play generated a lot of unpaid publicity. It is being broadcast on Turkish radio, numerous articles appeared in the press and it is being filmed incorporating some advice from a Turkish–Cypriot GP as evaluation had shown that advice from a doctor was deemed the most effective motivating action.

What might be the advantages of using drama as a method of smoking prevention? What are its limitations?

Skin cancer

The national priority has been to halt the year on year increase in the incidence of skin cancer by the year 2005. Each year in England, about 28,000 people develop skin cancers. Malignant melanoma occurs in all adult age groups and is curable if treated early, but often fatal if not detected. By far the greatest scope for reducing ill-health and disease caused by skin cancer is the prevention and early detection of malignant melanoma. The main risk factor, which also accounts for the increase in incidence in recent years, is the increased extent to which people are exposed, via the sun or sunbeds, to ultraviolet (UV) radiation.

Approaches to skin cancer prevention

The three key actions needed to halt the increased rates of skin cancer are:

- to increase the number of people who are aware of their own skin cancer risk factors;
- to persuade people at high risk to avoid excessive exposure to the sun and artificial sources of light, for themselves and their children, through the adoption of appropriate sun protection;
- to alter people's attitude to a tanned appearance.

Underlying these actions is the principle that prevention is as important an intervention as treatment. Primary prevention focusing on sensible exposure to the sun is more likely to be successful than discouraging exposure to the sun altogether. Information on the strength of UV radiation from the sun around noon, providing shade in public spaces, and encouraging the use of appropriate protective clothing such as loose cotton tee-shirts and sun hats are all important elements of a primary prevention campaign. The health promotion response has been to emphasize individual and especially parental responsibility for changing behaviour to reduce exposure. However, many other factors are also involved, and ignoring these other factors will reduce the effectiveness of health promotion interventions.

A ctivity

Common health promotion messages are:

- Wear sunhats.
- Wear protective clothing.
- Use sunscreen/sunblocks of appropriate strength.

How could health promotion address these other factors:

- Thinning of the ozone layer.
- Lack of shaded areas in school playgrounds.
- Attitudes which equate tanned skin with health.
- Outdoor workers who spend many hours unprotected in the sun.

Evidence of effective interventions

To date, there has been little evaluation of primary prevention in the UK, although studies in Sweden (Boldeman *et al.*, 1991) and Hawaii (King *et al.*, 1988) suggest that providing information about skin cancer can increase awareness about skin cancer and the intention to use sunscreen products. In the UK, the level of public awareness of the dangers of unprotected sunlight exposure is increasing. A wider range of more effective sunscreens (which filter out both UVB and

UVA radiation) are available and more widely used (assuming sales are a reliable indicator of use), although price is likely to be a barrier to use by those on a low income.

Secondary prevention (or early detection) of skin cancer, and in particular malignant melanoma, is important (DoH, 1993). Following an awareness raising campaign in 1985 there was an increase of 23% in the number of melanomas diagnosed in the first year of the campaign compared with the previous year. There was also a statistically significant fall in the average tumour thickness of melanomas (Doherty and Mackie, 1988). However, although this early detection programme seems to have been successful for women, no similar benefit has been shown to exist so far for men. There are difficulties with any secondary prevention programme. Such programmes generate considerable extra workload for general practitioners, dermatologists and pathologists; and the proportion of melanomas missed when using any kind of checklist is not yet known (Whitehead *et al.*, 1989; Graham-Brown *et al.*, 1990).

D What should be the balance of priorities between primary and secondary prevention of skin cancer?

Breast cancer

Breast cancer is the most important cause of premature deaths from cancer among women. Each year in England nearly 22,000 women are diagnosed as having breast cancer (1:14 women) and 13,000 women die from it. Advances in the treatment of breast cancer in recent years have meant less radical, mutilating surgery. The earlier breast cancer is treated the greater the chance of undergoing minimal surgery and the better the chances of success. The 1997 national target for breast cancer was:

■ To reduce the rate of breast cancer deaths among women invited for screening by at least 25% by the year 2000.

Approaches to breast cancer prevention

Although there have been advances in treatment, survival rates have improved only slightly. The search for a means of primary prevention therefore remains the focus of much research and debate. However primary prevention of breast cancer is problematic (Knight and Taylor, 1989; Taylor and Cudby, 1992a). Some of the risk factors such as early menstruation, late menopause and age at first full-term pregnancy are not open to intervention. The evidence for other risk factors such as use of oral contraceptives, obesity, excessive alcohol consumption, use of Hormone Replacement Therapy and the protective effect of breast feeding are less clear cut. Attention has therefore focused on secondary prevention and led to the establishment of a national Breast Cancer Screening Programme (NHSBSP). Women aged 50 to 64 are invited for

D Breast cancer incidence increases with age and most cases are found in women aged over 65 years. What rationale is there for restricting the NHS Breast Screening Programme (NHSBSP) to women aged 50 to 64?

screening every three years. Women over 64 need to request an appointment.

Limited resources mean that some form of targeting or rationing is seen as appropriate. The risk of breast cancer starts to increase in those aged over 50. Mammograms are also less sensitive in younger women with dense breast tissue. The cut-off at age 64 would appear to have more to do with ageism than epidemiology as the incidence is high in this older age group. Hence there are concerns that the way in which the breast screening service is organized is failing older women (Mullagh, 1996).

The success of the NHSBSP in reducing mortality from breast cancer in women over 50 is dependent on at least 70% uptake by eligible women (Cook *et al.*, 1989; Taylor and Cudby, 1992b). Increasing uptake is therefore a priority and the new Labour government has committed itself to addressing inequities in the screening programme. Improving the efficiency of the system which invites women for screening is also a key element. Careful checking of records and lists, active promotion of the NHSBSP to patients, and discussions with women who did not attend on their next visit to the practice have all been shown to have a powerful effect on uptake rates (Taylor, 1992). The following case study illustrates how Practice Nurses can increase uptake of the screening programme.

C ase study

The role of the practice nurse

Promoting breast screening in inner city areas can be a particular challenge. Health authorities send GP practices Prior Notification Lists which indicate women aged 50–64 who are eligible for screening. However, movement by patients in cities can mean such lists are not accurate and may be inflated by up to 30%. In larger practices over 500 patients may be listed. Some health authorities pay practices £50–170 to encourage them to check the Prior Notification Lists against practice registers.

Practice nurses, with the support of reception staff and the agreement of doctors and practice managers, are ideally placed to ensure these are correctly completed. Practice nurses whose practices achieve over 80% on cervical screening targets are likely to have well kept medical records and computer systems and to have fostered a positive approach to screening programmes amongst their patients.

In North London, an inner city practice achieved a previously unheard of 66% uptake for breast screening.

Several factors are likely to have contributed to this achievement – both individually and in combination:

- The commitment of the practice nurse, supported by reception staff, who checked every patient record against the Prior Notification List.

- The accurate patient database, with virtually no list inflation amongst screening age women.
- The easy accessibility of the Breast Screening Mobile – at a super-market site, in a main shopping area, close to the surgery.
- The fact some women were attending for screening during the breast awareness 'pink ribbon' month in October 1996.
- The availability in the practice of a multilingual photostory leaflet which reinforced the information included with the invitation to first screening.
- The existence of a Screening Facilitator to encourage and support primary care services.

Promoting the service to women through a range of community-based initiatives have been effective in encouraging and promoting positive attitudes to breast screening but do not necessarily have a great impact on uptake rates as shown in the following case study.

C ase study

Hairdressers for Health

Hairdressers for Health is an initiative set up in Kirkby with the initial intention of spreading positive health messages about the NHS Breast Screening Programme in the hope of encouraging attendance. The project was initiated by the Health Promotion Service of St Helens & Knowsley Community Health (NHS) Trust and has gained widespread local and national media interest which has reinforced positive messages in Kirkby.

The aims of Hairdressers for Health were to raise awareness of the NHSBSP and its benefits prior to and throughout the mobile screening unit's visit to Kirkby and to encourage positive attitudes towards screening. Specific objectives included ensuring that women had easy access to health information, received support and information from hairdressers and were in a position to make an informed choice about attending for breast screening. Additionally it was hoped that hair-dressers would act as a point of referral for further information and that discussing breast screening would act as a catalyst for discussion of other health issues. It was believed that working in partnership with hairdressers to promote the breast screening service would be effective because:

- Women aged 50 and over could be easily targeted.
- The hairdressing salon is an unthreatening environment to discuss what is a potentially sensitive issue.
- Hairdressers are often excellent communicators, spending the majority of their working day with members of the public, usually talking.
- This project was felt to be an ideal way of empowering local people to spread positive health messages within the community.

- Health is often routinely discussed in salons between hairdresser and client.
- Hairdressing salons are focal points in the community in Kirkby.

Initial visits to the twelve salons in Kirkby were made in February 1995 to assess their support and interest in being involved in preparation for mobile breast screening in April 1995. Eleven of the salons were enthusiastically supportive and wanted to be involved in encouraging women to go for breast screening. Each salon then received an individual briefing which covered the benefits of screening, what happened during the screening process, who was invited and why, an overview of treatment options and their role in offering information and encouragement. An information pack was produced which contained all the information discussed during the briefing and a section on "common questions women may ask you" for staff reference. In addition two posters were produced to raise awareness about the breast screening mobile coming to Kirkby and to let women know that their hairdressers had more information. Each salon also had leaflets to distribute.

During the initial 14-week period, 1800 leaflets were distributed. On average, each hairdresser (there were 31 participating stylists) spoke to 39 women per week about breast cancer/screening, reaching around 1200 women. All of the hairdressers said they felt the scheme had increased awareness about the importance of breast screening among their clients and had also increased their own awareness. From a sample of 60 women who completed questionnaires in the salons, 35% stated that they had previously heard about screening from the hairdressing salons. This was the most common venue for having seen publicity. Over 80% of the sample attended for breast screening which is much higher than the overall locality uptake and suggests that the initiative succeeded in encouraging women to attend for breast screening. This was supported by the finding that 31% of respondents specified that they had been encouraged to attend for breast screening by their hairdresser.

Hairdressers for Health is deemed to be a successful and innovative intervention winning several health awards. Five of the salons have continued to work with the health promotion service on a range of other health issues. These include encouraging non-attendees to make another appointment; assistance with research into non-attendance (not yet complete); promotion of National No Smoking Day and publicizing the counselling service offered by the Health Promotion Service for people wanting to stop; and promoting key messages concerning cervical cancer screening. In four of the salons prize money awarded to the health promotion service for the Hairdressers for Health initiative has been used to install Health Information Systems. Televisions have been wall mounted in the salons and every two months a new health promotion video is shown which ensures there are ongoing health messages on a variety of topics. Yet although the original aims and objectives of the Hairdressers for Health were successfully met and there has been continued commitment from all the hairdressers the overall impact on the breast screening uptake rate was negligible (59% compared with 58%).

- How would you respond to criticism that "Hairdressers for Health" is an example of a creeping medicalization of people's private lives?
- Why might eligible women refuse the offer of breast screening?

Limitations of breast cancer screening

What has been called "cancerphobia" is one explanation for a reluctance to attend for screening. Although most women consider breast cancer to be a serious threat to health, for some that threat appears so great that it becomes a fear. The beliefs that

- cancer is not curable;
- that X-rays in themselves are harmful;
- that any treatment is painful and not necessarily successful;
- that the major risk factor for breast cancer is genetic inheritance;

may all inhibit women from going for screening. In addition as in all screening programmes, coverage is not uniform (DoH, 1996). Poverty and deprivation are associated with lower take-up rates. This might reflect different beliefs and attitudes towards cancer, but it also reflects different perceptions of the accessibility of the service offered. The individual costs and benefits of attending for breast screening are affected by many factors including:

- transport costs;
- provision of care services if a woman is a carer;
- language (is the service in the woman's home language?);
- whether time is needed off work.

Breast awareness

The NHSBSP is an important programme for targeted women. However, the extent of breast cancer means that all women should be encouraged to report any signs or symptoms of breast disease (Taylor and Cudby, 1993). The Department of Health first issued advice on breast self-examination in 1989. More recently, the concept of breast awareness has been advocated. Breast awareness refers to "women's ability to distinguish for themselves the difference between normal and abnormal changes in their breasts". This is different from breast self-examination which was presented as a self-administered screening test and criticized for its lack of specificity (i.e. many women found lumps but few were actually cancerous) and for suggesting that self-examination was an alternative to mammography. Since over 90% of breast cancers are found by women themselves (CMO, 1991), the Department of Health suggest there is scope for increasing the breast awareness of women under 50 and encouraging women to report any symptoms early.

Breast awareness does not reduce the chances of getting breast cancer. It actually increases the chances of finding a lump and identifying cancer. On the one hand, it may lessen the consequences of breast cancer (if tumours are found earlier and treated sooner) but on the other hand it may raise anxiety. A successful breast awareness campaign will increase demands on a range of health practitioners to further investigate unusual symptoms.

Cervical cancer

The national target for cervical cancer is:

- To reduce the incidence of invasive cancer from 15 per 100,000 population in 1986 to no more than 12 per 100,000 in the year 2000.

Cervical cancer, unlike breast cancer, is a totally preventable disease. Despite this, in England, cervical cancer occurs in 3500 women each year and over 1500 die from it, the majority of whom have never had a cervical smear test (McKie, 1993). The number of positive smears has risen in the last decade and the majority of these are in women under 35, suggesting that without screening the mortality rate would be higher (Chomet and Chomet, 1989). Suspected risk factors include genetic causes, smoking, age of first sexual intercourse, number of sexual partners (of women and their partners), partners who work in dusty occupations, personal hygiene, a lowered immune response and a range of viruses (especially Human Papillomavirus). Protective factors include the use of barrier methods of contraception (condoms, caps), celibacy, lesbianism and male circumcision.

Secondary prevention focuses on the early detection and treatment of pre-cancer changes in the cervix through the establishment of a fully computerized national call/recall cervical screening programme (NHSCSP) for all women aged 20–64. The earlier pre-cancerous changes in the cervix are treated the greater the chance of success. Evidence from other countries suggests that well organized and co-ordinated programmes are successful in reducing the incidence of invasive cancer and, in addition, can achieve a significant reduction in cervical cancer deaths, although this is dependent on reaching a high proportion of targeted women (for example, 80% of women aged 25–59 were screened in Iceland (Singer & Szarewski, 1988)).

D The following have been identified as indicators of possible breast cancer:

- Any unusual change in the outline, shape or size of the breast.
- Puckering or dimpling of the skin.
- A lump in the breast or armpit.
- Any flaking of the skin or discharge (including blood) from the nipple.
- Any unusual pain or discomfort.

What problems might be associated with an effective breast awareness campaign?

12 Sexual health promotion

Jo Mussen, Jennie Naidoo and Jane Wills

Key points

- Defining sexual health.
- National health strategy.
- Sexual health promotion.
- Approaches to HIV reduction and prevention:
  - □ changing behaviour;
  - □ personal strategies for health.

Overview

This chapter looks at sexual health, with particular reference to reducing the spread of the Human Immune Deficiency Virus (HIV). Sexual health, in common with mental health, is a broadly contested concept. This chapter begins by exploring what is meant by sexual health and acknowledges the social context within which sexual health is understood. The difficulties of achieving a public consensus about sexual health have resulted in the dominance of medical definitions concentrating on the prevention of ill-health arising from sexual activity (e.g. prevention of teenage pregnancy, prevention of sexually transmitted diseases). This chapter reviews some of the approaches that have been taken to HIV prevention. It focuses, in particular, on client-centred strategies and discusses why endorsing a principle of empowerment can be particularly difficult when working to reduce HIV. Two case studies are presented of "personal strategies for health" in a genito-urinary medicine (GUM) clinic and the production of a written information resource for gay men – "Thinking it Through".

Introduction

The term sexual health has many contrasting definitions, which are influenced by beliefs about concepts such as health and sex. Definitions may range from a focus on the clinical causes of physical ill-health, such as infections, to a celebration of pleasure.

R

Consider the following definitions of sexual health. Which comes closest to your own and why?

- The integration of the physical, emotional, intellectual and social aspects of sexual being, in ways that are enriching and that enhance personality, communication and love (WHO, 1974, quoted in HEA,

1994:4). WHO identifies three elements which should inform discussions of sexuality and sexual health:

(a) the capacity to enjoy and express sexuality without guilt or shame in fulfilling, emotional relationships;

(b) the capacity to control fertility;

(c) freedom from disorders which compromise health and sexual or reproductive function.

- A state of physical and psychological well-being characterized by the absence of sexually transmitted diseases and unintended pregnancies, due to freely considered, informed choices on personal relationships and sexual practices (Kapila, 1990).

- An integral part of overall health, not restricted to the avoidance of STDs and HIV/AIDS . . . sexual health requires the enjoyment of free choice, expression and responsibility with particular regard to the prevention of the transmission of STDs and HIV (Curtis, 1992).

Do these definitions impact equally on men and women? On heterosexual and homosexual people?

There is considerable evidence that gender is an important factor affecting sexual health. "The differential power of men and women is evident in most sexual intercourse as it is in the wider context of male–female relations" (Doyal, 1995:62). Women's capacity to enjoy and express their sexuality is limited by the fundamentally unequal relationship between men and women. Women may have to negotiate about fertility and safer sex and may be under threat from violence, harassment or abuse. A survey of young women's sexual attitudes concludes that "For a young woman to insist on the use of a condom for her own safety requires resisting the constraints and opposing the construction of intercourse as a man's natural pleasure and a woman's natural duty" (Thomson and Holland, 1995:24).

Homosexuality remains a less socially valued and more discriminated against sexual identity, compared to heterosexuality. Activities which heterosexuals take for granted such as public recognition and acceptance of their sexual partners can be problematic for homosexuals. The rights of homosexuals are proscribed by law, e.g. the age of consent for homosexuals is 18 compared to 16 for heterosexuals; homosexuals are refused entry into the armed forces.

The national health strategy

The "Health of the Nation" strategy on HIV/AIDS and sexual health is based on an illness model. While it acknowledges that "good personal and sexual relationships can actively promote health and well being", it goes on to add that "on the other hand, sexual activity can sometimes lead to unwanted pregnancies, ill health or disease" (DoH, 1992:92). It is easy to understand why sexual health promotion refers more commonly to the prevention of sexually transmitted infections and unwanted pregnancies than to sexual well-being and fulfilment. There is considerable public controversy concerning the acceptable or desirable boundaries of sexual activity. By contrast, there is a consensus that reducing the harmful effects of sexual activity is desirable.

Activity

> Staff at a centre for young people with learning difficulties want to provide sex education within the personal education programme. The young people have expressed an interest. Some parents argue that such a programme is inappropriate and could lead to precocious and/or promiscuous sexual activity. Other parents argue it would help their children protect themselves from unwanted sexual attention or abuse. Centre staff argue that their clients have a right to sexually fulfilling relationships and activities.
>
> If you were manager of the centre, how would you respond to these different views? What action would you take?

The "Health of the Nation" strategy included targets relating to teenage pregnancies, the availability of family planning services and a reduction in the incidence of sexually transmitted diseases and HIV infection. However most health promotion work has tended to focus on HIV, due to the existence of ring-fenced funding, the appointment of HIV Prevention Co-ordinators and major national campaigns. This chapter therefore concentrates on HIV prevention initiatives.

The following three criteria were used to identify national priorities for health improvement in the "Health of the Nation" strategy:

D According to these criteria, to what extent does HIV prevention warrant inclusion as a target?

- that there was a major cause of premature death or avoidable ill-health;
- that effective interventions were possible;
- that it was possible to set objectives and targets.

HIV clearly meets the first criterion. In one of the progress reports on "The Health of the Nation" it is stated that "AIDS has come to rank amongst the top dozen leading causes of life years lost in this country for people under 65; that is for people who form the bulk of the workforce" (DoH, 1995:91). Later in this chapter we discuss the difficulties of designing interventions to promote sexual health and the evidence that exists for effective interventions. Turning to the third criterion, it is difficult to set targets for improvements in sexual health. This would certainly be the case if a definition of sexual well-being were used and is still difficult if HIV infection is targeted, given the timelag between infection, diagnosis and the development of symptoms. HIV had been excluded from the consultative Green Paper preceding "The Health of the Nation" as it was felt that specific, measurable targets could not be set. Rates of gonorrhoea infection and drug injecting were then identified as proxy targets for reducing the transmission of HIV, while it was felt that attempts to meet the target for teenage pregnancies would contribute to healthy sexual behaviour (Thin, 1993). It could be argued that proxy markers such as the incidence of gonorrhoea are of limited relevance. The incidence of gonorrhoea was dropping already at the time of publishing the White Paper and, in the opinion of many clinicians, the target was achievable without any added intervention.

Sexual health promotion

D How feasible is it to set targets for sexual health? The Health of the Nation sets targets to:

- reduce the incidence of gonorrhoea;
- reduce the rate of conceptions amongst the under 16s;
- reduce the percentage of injecting drug users who report sharing equipment.

Are these targets relevant to the WHO definition of sexual health outlined on page 238?

Sexual health behaviour differs from other health-related behaviours, such as eating an unhealthy diet or drinking alcohol, in that when infection is present an individual's behaviour may have a direct, immediate and drastic effect on their sexual partner's health. This has always been the case, but in the past bacterial STDS like gonorrhoea could be treated and cured, while other chronic viral conditions like genital warts or herpes could be extremely unpleasant but not fatal. The HIV epidemic has engendered a far greater sense of urgency than has existed since the widespread availability of antibiotics. This sense of urgency has resulted in an understandable desire to encourage individuals to change their sexual behaviour, in order to protect themselves and their partners from HIV. However there has tended to be a narrow focus on individual sexual behaviour, out of the context of the many influences on sexual health and behaviour. It could be argued that this in turn has hampered the development of effective interventions in sexual health promotion, particularly within the statutory sector. Interventions have tended to rely on a "top-down" approach, giving information and targeting individual behaviour. The Key Area Handbook (DoH, 1993:42) reflects this approach in its three aims for health promotion work to reduce HIV:

- To improve levels of knowledge and awareness about HIV among the general population and specific targeted groups.
- To encourage people to adopt healthy or safer patterns of sexual behaviour.
- To encourage people who may be at continued risk to modify and sustain changes in their sexual behaviour.

Sexual health and sexuality, while higher on the political agenda than they were prior to HIV, remain politically sensitive subjects characterized by mixed messages:

- Information campaigns aimed at the general population to inform about HIV and ways individuals can protect themselves have been acceptable, but detailed discussion of sexual activities and pleasures, especially by gay men and lesbians, is still a very sensitive issue.

■ It is hoped to reduce the rate of teenage pregnancy, yet sex education is present on the National Curriculum to a very limited extent, with the emphasis on biology and physiology. Beyond this statutory requirement sex education is the responsibility of school governing bodies which "gives schools a good deal of flexibility to take account of local circumstances and the views of parents" (DoH, 1992:99).

■ Part of Government strategy is to take into account social, legal and ethical issues "fostering a climate of understanding and compassion, discouraging discrimination, and safeguarding confidentiality" (DoH, 1992:98). Yet in 1995 an attempt to lower the age of consent for gay men to that for heterosexuals failed and one of the effects of the 1996 Asylum Act is to deter refugees from accessing health services, because of fear of enquiry into their immigration status.

It is difficult to target messages for sexual health because:

R Why do you think it is particularly difficult to design interventions to promote sexual health?

■ Each person has a different attitude to their sexual health influenced by their needs, self-esteem, confidence and their peer norms.

■ Sexual behaviour does not occur in isolation, but involves at least one other person and is therefore also affected by their needs and values.

■ There is a lack of information about people's knowledge and behaviour. Many aspects of sexual behaviour are considered to be private and taboo. In the past this has led to abandoning plans for a national survey on sexual behaviour (Wellings *et al.*, 1994). Research into sexual behaviour is beset by problems of what language to use to describe sex and relationships.

■ Again, because there is no universally accepted language with which to describe sex, it is difficult to identify effective means of communicating messages about sexual health to a public audience.

■ The political ideology of the New Right in the UK over the last eighteen years has been to establish a moral climate of family values (Durham, 1991) which has made more invisible much homosexual and bisexual activity and made the targeting of messages to men who have sex with men particularly difficult (see Chapter 5 for a discussion on the changing response to HIV/AIDS in public policy).

D The following statements from health promotion practitioners reflect a range of views about the purposes of sexual health promotion. How does this diversity make it difficult to promote sexual health?

- "Sex education isn't about providing information – it is about communicating clear moral standards which state that sexual activity belongs within a monogamous marriage" (School head teacher).
- "Our clients come with a specific disease which they want cured. Our job is to treat the disease and prevent its spread, not to moralize or advise clients on their lifestyle" (GUM Health Adviser).
- "Sexual activity is a very private affair. I wouldn't dream of raising the subject unless a client did first – and even then to be honest I would find it difficult. Discussing contraceptive methods is fine, but anything else . . ." (Practice Nurse).
- "People need the space to discuss their sexuality, be validated with regard to their choices and behaviour" (Volunteer Counsellor).
- "The message sounds simple – use a condom every time – but we know it's not that simple, or realistic" (Health Promotion Specialist).

Approaches to HIV reduction and prevention

Chapter 5 discussed the concept of targeting and the categories of risk adopted in health promotion. HIV prevention work has targeted:

- **Risky behaviours**
  e.g.   by organizing STD testing and condom distribution for sex workers;
  needle exchange schemes;
  by organizing erotic sex workshops to encourage non-penetrative sexual activity.
- **Risk groups**
  e.g.   men who have sex with men;
  injecting drug users;
  African communities;
  sex workers;
  prisoners.

Interventions to reduce the spread of HIV can thus be categorized into those which seek to:

(a) reduce the risk of infection through information and education about safer sex;
(b) empower sexually active people by improving self-esteem, developing assertiveness and negotiation skills; and
(c) develop the strength of particular communities.

Changing sexual behaviour

One dilemma for health promotion is deciding the message to be adopted to promote sexual health. Reducing the spread of infection has been deemed the major priority of the "Health of the Nation" strategy. However, reducing risk would mean one of the following:

- the regular use of condoms possibly together with other methods of contraception (none of which are 100% reliable);
- insisting on a sexual health screen, including HIV test, followed by treatment of any infections before sex with any new sexual partner (although chronic viral conditions such as herpes, warts or HIV are not curable and sex is generally regarded as a spontaneous act);
- monogamy or sexual abstinence for life.

It is obviously unrealistic to expect people to adopt these behaviours. Even the simple message always to use a condom is inappropriate when perceptions of risk are low as they are among most heterosexuals, particularly those over 35 (HEA, 1994). Thus many interventions which seek to effect behavioural change have been shown to increase knowledge but have had little effect on attitudes and behaviour (e.g. McEwan and Bhopal, 1991).

There is now considerable evidence that the relative success of promoting safer sex messages to the gay community has been through the actions of the community itself rather than any health education campaign or intervention:

"The history of the last decade shows that there is a clear correlation between the widespread adoption of safer sex and the existence of a confident and supportive gay affirmative culture providing grassroots community education. By contrast there is no correlation recorded anywhere in the world between the widespread adoption of safer sex and the attempt to impose warnings from above using individualistic models of behaviour change"

(Rooney and Scott, 1992:51).

The work of Kelly *et al.* (1992) in the USA has been influential in showing that community interventions are effective in changing behaviour. In this research an intervention took place in gay bars of four cities, with four other cities as matched controls. Gay men identified as popular opinion leaders (or "gay heroes") were trained to give positive messages about safer sex to their peers. The intervention resulted in a decrease in the proportion of men who had unprotected anal sex (from 33% to 25%). In the UK, Gay Men Fighting AIDS is a community mobilization project which aims to encourage gay men to become peer educators in the community, recreating the early grass roots response to the epidemic.

Going beyond information and individual behaviour to empowerment

Sexual health involves more than merely the absence of disease and therefore to promote sexual health is to address broader influences on sexual health. It is also pragmatic to do so, in that it may be more possible to change some of the factors which influence behaviour than to change behaviour directly.

Sexual health promotion can attempt to target the many other factors which affect sexual health including:

- behaviour in its broader social context, i.e. recognizing the influence of peer norms, empowering/supporting communities in prevention efforts;
- legislation and policy, e.g. age of consent for gay sex, sex education in schools;
- access to appropriate information and services, e.g. provision of condoms including those for anal sex, contraception, advice and treatment for STDs.

Tones and Tilford (1994) have described empowerment as central to the ideology and practice of health promotion. To work towards empowerment is to facilitate people's choices by providing support and enabling skills. In one-to-one client encounters it is the client who raises issues of concern to them and the only outcomes for the health promoter are those of raising self-esteem, feelings of perceived control, and decision making skills. The practitioner does not have a pre-determined outcome of getting the client to change their behaviour. Instead of giving standard information on using a condom without regard to individual circumstances, the health promoter may suggest small steps to reduce risks which people can build into their lives, rather than proscribing certain activities (Hart, 1993).

Person-centred advice on risk reduction could be called a "personal strategies" approach to sexual health promotion. This approach has been used for some time by the Health Promotion Service in Camden and Islington and by other services and individuals (see, for example, Hart, 1993 and Wellings et al., 1994). The approach is based on the idea that there are many possible strategies which an individual may adopt to reduce the risk of HIV, other STDs or pregnancy. The context of a person's life and relationships needs to be investigated and acknowledged if they are to be supported in developing their own personal strategy for sexual health.

Rosser et al. (1993) suggest that the goal at this stage of the epidemic is to promote long-term maintenance of safer sex among homosexually active men. They suggest that to achieve this goal, individualized methods of intervention are necessary.

Abraham and Sheeran (1993) argue that most health promotion interventions target individuals, not couples, and focus on individual beliefs rather than skills of assertion, negotiation and problem solving. They suggest that much sexual activity is not open to negotiation

D "The moral imperative (of empowerment approaches) is essentially voluntarisitic and utilitarian: the guideline is that people's decisions are ethical provided that they do not harm others and do not impinge on others' freedom to act" (Tones, 1995). What ethical dilemmas are presented for the health promoter in adopting an empowerment/ "personal strategies" approach to HIV?

and that sexual social skills training especially for young people "would not only aim to bring about dramatic changes in the management of sexual relations but a radical shift in power relations between men and women. This will certainly involve a social transformatory approach to health promotion" (Abraham and Sheeran, 1993:250).

Increasingly, health promoters who work with drug users adopt a harm minimization approach which accepts that people may use drugs but they can be given information and skills to reduce their risks from so doing. Health promoters working to reduce HIV are similarly accepting that risk *reduction* rather than risk *elimination* may be a more realistic objective. This may mean accepting the reality of open relationships among gay men or that some men may choose to have unsafe sex. For example, if unprotected anal sex is something which a person enjoys, could it form part of a step-by-step risk reduction strategy for sexual health? If so, a number of ethical issues and implications for working practice would need to be considered. These include:

- whether that person is in a relationship;
- whether that relationship is monogamous;
- whether there are any rules for sex outside the relationship;
- whether there are contingency plans if those rules are not followed;
- and probably most importantly the HIV/STD status of that person and their partner(s).

C ase study

Thinking it Through – *a resource for gay men*

For many gay men in the UK, gay newspapers, magazines, leaflets and posters have been the most important source of information about safer sex (Davies *et al.*, 1993). Most campaigns and resources adopt a uniform message of safer sex. For example a list of resources produced by the Health Education Authority to support its work in reducing HIV among gay men includes a range of posters of gay men with the slogan "choose safer sex". As McKevitt *et al.* (1994) point out, if media are to represent and speak to the diversity of gay and bisexual men then it needs different messages which move beyond information giving to empowering change. A more sophisticated approach to written materials can be found in the booklet *Thinking it Through* which was launched in 1996.

This booklet was developed jointly by the Health Promotion and GUM Services of Camden and Islington NHS Trust and by Sigma Research as a response to the growing evidence that most unprotected sexual activity by gay men takes place in relationships rather than in casual sex (e.g. Keogh *et al.*, 1995). A sexual lifestyles survey at the Gay Pride festival in 1994 found that many gay men in relationships see unprotected sex as an expression of their emotional commitment to their partner (Hickson *et al.*, 1994). Alongside this evidence were reports from the genito-urinary medicine clinic that many gay men were coming for HIV tests in order to make decisions on whether to use condoms in their relationship (Maguire, 1997).

The booklet addresses the issues of non condom use among gay men, suggesting that the decision not to use condoms is one that needs "thinking through". The complex issues of sexual decision making are discussed, e.g.

- If one partner is positive, do they have a greater "responsibility " to use condoms than their partner who may be negative or not know their sero status?
- Should gay men in relationships always be tested before giving up using condoms?
- Should two positive men still use condoms?
- How can two negative men protect themselves and stay negative?

The aim was to explore the issues of sex within gay relationships with the aim of reducing the risks of unsafe sex and to enable gay partners to develop their personal strategy for health. The resource was extensively piloted in five cities and with focus groups made up of different target audiences, e.g. men with HIV, young men and older men.

D In 1986 Farrant and Russell observed that there is "an almost universal and unquestioned dictate of health education that a publication targeted at the general public should be short and simple with a reading age no higher than that of a tabloid newspaper" (Farrant and Russell, 1986:37). Do you agree?

The piloting of *Thinking it Through* resulted in a booklet of 40 pages with a readability age of twelve years. It differs from the prescriptive style of communication evident in many sexual health publications which are intended to "sell" a blanket safer sex message to a heterogeneous audience (see Chapter 5 for a detailed discussion of marketing strategies in health promotion). The booklet has been produced at a relatively low cost and ease of production and can be widely distributed through places accessed by gay men, e.g. clubs and pubs, gyms and GUM clinics.

Genito-urinary medicine service

The genito-urinary medicine service consists of a nationwide network of free clinics which predate the NHS. Clients can refer themselves to clinics and all information on clients, including HIV test results, is treated in strictest confidence, as required by an Act of Parliament in 1917.

The GUM Service has always had an important public health role to play in the control of sexually transmitted diseases (STDs). However the past emphasis on such curable, bacterial STDs as chlamydia, gonorrhoea and syphilis has meant that this role could be fulfilled by following a purely medical model in dealing with clients,

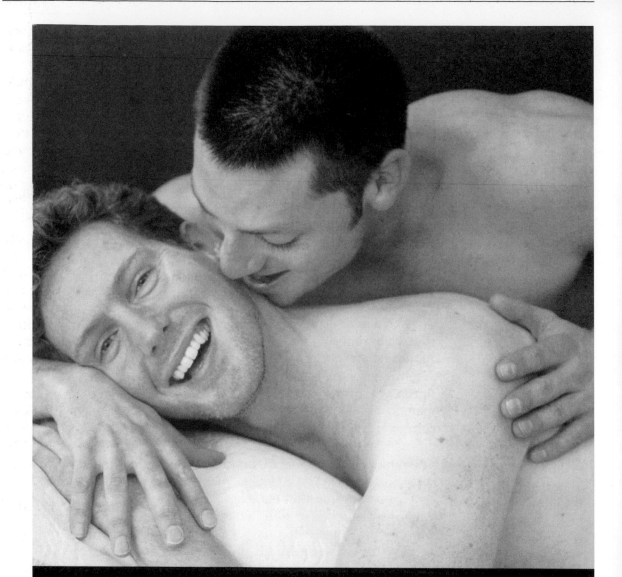

thinking **it** through
a new approach to
sex, relationships & HIV
for gay men

concentrating on diagnosis, treatment and partner notification. It was not essential for the Service to consider either the broad area of sexuality or the details of sexual activities (Pillaye, 1994).

In the past decade there has been a shift of emphasis in the workload of GUM clinics away from bacterial STDs towards the chronic viral infections of herpes, genital warts and HIV. This has made the public health role of clinics more complex because while such infections can be diagnosed and treated, they cannot be cured. There has also been a substantial increase in the number of clients seeking advice, counselling and HIV tests (Bentley and Adler, 1993). The GUM Service has consequently moved from being a "Cinderella" specialism to relatively "well funded, high status work" (Silverman, 1990: 197). The nature of the work has also changed – clients want to discuss other issues around sexual health (e.g. sexual orientation, sexual function). There is therefore a need for GUM staff to look beyond simply encouraging and supporting behaviour change and preventing the spread of infection to partners, to broader promotion of sexual health. This emphasis on looking at sexual lifestyles represents the possibility of a fundamental paradigm shift, away from a traditional medical model towards a more person centred approach to health care and health promotion.

The changing role of GUM clinics was recognized in a Government report on their workloads (DoH, 1988) which, among other recommendations, suggested that all clinics should have health advisers and facilities to provide comprehensive counselling. The work of this report was taken further in a study of work roles and responsibilities in GUM clinics which recommended that:

> "the role of GUM clinic staff, not only in controlling the spread of infection but also in creating and maintaining 'sexual health' in the population by means of education and health promotion . . . should be developed"
>
> (Allen and Hogg, 1993:224).

The GUM Service offers an ideal opportunity for interventions to promote sexual health. It is a unique statutory service, in that by attending the Service its clients are identifying themselves as at risk of STDs. Elsewhere it is notoriously difficult to identify individuals at risk within the population and targeting, is by necessity, quite crude. Attendance at a GUM clinic involves the client in one-to-one contact with a health professional where it is not only necessary but accepted as such that details of sexual activities are discussed.

The nature of the client group not only presents GUM staff with an opportunity for sexual health promotion, but also makes it essential to grasp this opportunity. This is especially true in London, where a recent survey found that 7.4% of men and 6.7% of women reported attending a GUM clinic in the last five years, a higher proportion than

Figure 12.1 Thinking it Through *booklet (opposite). Reproduced with kind permission of Camden and Islington Community Health Services NHS Trust.*

elsewhere in the country (Wellings *et al.*, 1994:298). The authors comment that these figures may well be an underestimate of clinic attendance, due to possible under-reporting. The survey finds a strong association between increased risk, in terms of the number of sexual partners, and increased likelihood of GUM clinic attendance. The authors conclude that:

> "This finding indicates that a high proportion of those at risk of STD and HIV are attending STD clinics and emphasises the importance of these health service settings for assisting individuals in risk reduction strategies"
>
> (Wellings *et al.*, 1994:320).

However, Johnson *et al.* (1994) point out that more than 80% of those surveyed who had had five or more heterosexual partners in the last five years had not attended a GUM clinic. This indicates that, in common with much of the health service, GUM clinics are viewed as relevant to diseases, rather than to health: people do not yet think in terms of a sexual health check up. This means that there are further opportunities for the GUM Service to contact those at risk of STDs "either through community approaches or greater accessibility" (Johnson *et al.*, 1994).

Case study

Training for GUM staff

In Camden & Islington a multidisciplinary working party, The Sexual Health Promotion Group, was set up (French and George, 1994) with the aim of assessing the extent of sexual health promotion in the GUM service and of making recommendations to enhance and improve current strategies.

Several key questions arose:

- Who is responsible for sexual health promotion in a GUM clinic – doctors, nurses or health advisers?
- Should sexual health promotion be part of every consultation?
- How should discussions about for example, safer sex or the prevention of transmission of warts, be approached?
- How could an area as broad as sexual health be broached in a busy clinic with time-limited consultations?
- What skills are necessary to be a sexual health promoter?

The working party made a number of recommendations, among them that doctors should routinely raise prevention with all new patients. This is because doctors see all patients new to the service. So by doctors routinely raising prevention, no patient will "slip through the net", that is attend the service without being given an opportunity to discuss their strategy for prevention. Secondly this recommendation ensures a high profile for prevention in the service, both for staff and for patients. To support this recommendation, it was also recommended that all medical staff receive training in communication skills.

The training was based on the following model of one-to-one sexual health promotion. It is important to have a model to give a practical framework to work within when there is very little time available.

$$
\boxed{\begin{array}{c}\text{Information and}\\\text{concerns from patient:}\\\text{Set in context of}\\\text{gender, sexuality,}\\\text{relationships etc.}\end{array}}\times\boxed{\begin{array}{c}\text{Information and}\\\text{questions from doctor:}\\\text{Responding to context}\\\text{of patient}\end{array}}=\boxed{\begin{array}{c}\text{Developing/refining}\\\text{"personal strategy" for}\\\text{sexual health}\end{array}}
$$

This model envisages the process of health promotion as two-way, with the expert input of the doctor (or nurse or health adviser) responding to, and varying, according to the concerns and the context of the patient. Both inputs may be necessary to develop or refine a patient's personal strategy for sexual health.

If this model is accepted, how do we then define what is expected of each individual doctor? The working party made a recommendation outlining certain minimum standards of practice. This said that all doctors should be able to:

- evaluate current sexual behaviour;
- advise about risks attached to different sexual activities;
- help patients reflect on their own personal situation;
- encourage them to make changes which will reduce risk;
- identify whether there is a need for referral or further discussion with another member of staff.

A two-day participative course in communication skills and sexual health was designed and has since been run twice a year, to cater for all medical staff in the service. It focused on a range of skills. The skills of closed questioning, checking what is already known or understood and giving information correspond to the first steps in the medical consultation. These are skills in which doctors are already well versed. However, other skills were new for some medical staff. These skills include open questioning, listening, being positive about achievements, recognizing distress or difficulty and giving advice and encouragement. The training also focused on referral to other staff and agencies. This is a crucial skill in that, while doctors can follow a model of good practice, there are limitations on how much they can achieve in the time available.

Activity

This case study illustrates how a systematic planned approach can increase opportunities for sexual health promotion in an identified setting. What aspects of this initiative could be transferred to other settings, e.g.

- a primary healthcare setting;
- a workplace occupational health service;
- a school health service.

Conclusion

This chapter has explored the concept of sexual health promotion and in particular has identified the difference between the prevention of sexual ill-health and the promotion of sexual health. The promotion of sexual health or well-being is fraught with problems because there is no public consensus about what these terms mean in practice, or the boundaries separating acceptable and unacceptable sexual activities. By contrast, preventing or reducing sexual activity is viewed as a legitimate practice belonging to medical practitioners.

National priorities for sexual health therefore focus, not surprisingly, on reducing the rate of sexually transmitted diseases and unwanted pregnancies. Whilst the narrow medical focus of these targets may be criticized, they have proved useful in stimulating a broader range of activities, illustrated by the two case studies discussed earlier.

The challenge for health promoters is to extend sexual health programmes beyond the prevention of the ill-health effects of sexual activity. This chapter has shown how a concern for empowerment and participation can be incorporated into programmes with a more traditional remit of prevention. However, the chapter also shows how sexual health is not equally accessible to all, irrespective of age, sexual orientation and identity or gender. Thus a focus on empowering individuals to sexual health whether it be through information, the learning of skills or sexual work without recognizing the importance of the social context is unlikely to be effective.

Further discussion

■   What are the advantages and disadvantages of medically defined prevention targets?
■   What aims can be identified for sexual health promotion (as distinct from prevention of sexual ill-health)? Can these aims be defined as targets?

Recommended reading

■   Aggleton P, Davies PM and Hart G (eds) (1990) *AIDS: Individual, policy and cultural dimensions*, London, Falmer Press.
    A review of AIDS policy which raises many of the issues discussed here but which is slightly dated.

■   Davies PM, Hickson FCI, Weatherburn P and Hunt AJ (1993) *Sex, Gay Men and AIDS*, London, Falmer Press.
    An historical overview of health promotion responses to the HIV epidemic in the UK with particular reference to issues of the de-gaying of HIV.

- Doyal L, Naidoo J and Wilton T (eds) (1994) *AIDS: setting a feminist agenda*, Basingstoke, Taylor and Francis.
This identifies the implications of the HIV/AIDS experience for women in the UK and presents an overview of the important issues raised for feminist theory and practice.

- Evans B, Sandberg S and Watson S (eds) (1992) *Working where the risks are: issues in HIV prevention*, London, Health Education Authority.
An authoritative discussion of the issues relating to HIV prevention which includes chapters on working with gay men, sex education for young people and working with ethnic minority communities.

References

Abraham C and Sheeran P (1993) "In search of a psychology of safer sex promotion: beyond beliefs and texts", *Health Education Research* **8**(2), 245–54.

Allen I and Hogg D (1993) *Work Roles and Responsibilities in Genitourinary Medicine Clinics*, London, PSI.

Bentley C and Adler M (1993) "G.U.M., AIDS and the NHS Act: will contracting arrangements lead to contracted services?" *Genitourinary Medicine*, **67**, 10–14.

Curtis M (ed.) (1992) *Promoting sexual health*, London, BMA Foundation for AIDS.

Davies PM, Hickson FCI, Weatherburn P and Hunt AJ (1993) *Sex, Gay Men and AIDS*, London, Falmer Press.

Department of Health (1988) *Report of working group to examine workloads in GUM clinics: the Monks Report*, London, HMSO.

Department of Health (1992) *The Health of the Nation*, London, HMSO.

Department of Health (1993) *Key Area Handbook: HIV/AIDS and Sexual Health*, London, DoH.

Department of Health (1995) *Fit for the Future: Second Progress Report of the Health of the Nation,* London, DoH.

Doyal L (1995) *What makes women sick: gender and the political economy of health*, Basingstoke, Macmillan.

Durham M (1991) *Sex and Politics: the family and morality in the Thatcher Years*, Basingstoke, Macmillan Education.

Farrant W and Russell J (1986) *The Politics of Health Information*, University of London.

French P and George V (1994) *Developing a Sexual Health Promotion Strategy in the GUM Service: Report of the Sexual Health Promotion Group*, London, Camden and Islington Community Health Services NHS Trust.

Hart G (1993) "Safer Sex: A Paradigm Revisited", in P. Aggleton *et al.* (eds) *AIDS: Facing the Second Decade*, London, Falmer Press.

HEA (1994) *Health Update no. 4 Sexual Health*, London, Health Education Authority.

Hickson FCI, Beardsall S, Broderick P *et al.* (1994) *Gay men's Sex Survey at Pride 94*, London, Project Sigma.

Kapila M (1990) "Improving sexual health", *AIDS Dialogue*, **7**, 3–4.

Kelly JA, St Lawrence JS, Stevenson LY *et al.* (1992) "Community AIDS/HIV risk reduction: the effects of endorsements by popular people in three cities" *American Journal of Public Health*, **82**, 1483–89.

Keogh P, Beardsall S, Hickson FCI and Reid DS (1995) *Sexual Health Needs of HIV-positive gay and bisexual men*, London, Project Sigma.

Johnson AM, Wadsworth, J, Wellings K and Field J (1994) *Characteristics of GUM clinic attenders from the National Survey of Sexual Attitudes and Lifestyles*, Liverpool, paper to the MSSVD conference, 12–15 May.

McEwan R and Bhopal R (1991) *HIV/AIDS health promotion for young people: a review of theory, principles and practice*, London, Health Education Authority.

McKevitt C, Warwick I and Aggleton P (1994) *Towards good practice*, London, Health Education Authority.

Maguire M (1997) Team leader Sexual Health Promotion Camden and Islington Community Health Services NHS Trust, *Personal communication*.

Pillaye J (1994) *Sexual health promotion in GUM clinics*, London, Health Education Authority.

Rooney M and Scott P (1992) "Working where the risks are: health promotion interventions for men who have sex with men", in Evans B, Sandberg S and Watson S (eds) *Working where the risks are: issues in HIV prevention*, London, Health Education Authority.

Rosser BRS, Coleman E and Ohmans P (1993) "Safer sex maintenance and reduction of unsafe sex among homosexually active men: a new therapeutic approach", *Health Education Research* **8**(1), 19–34.

Silverman D (1990) "The Social Organisation of HIV Counselling", in Aggleton P *et al.* (eds) *AIDS: Individual, Cultural and Policy Perspectives*, London, Falmer Press.

Thin RN (1993) "Health of the Nation: a way forward in sexual health", *Journal of Royal Society of Medicine*, **113**(1), 40–42.

Thomson R and Holland J (1994) "Young women and safer (hetero) sex: context, constraints and strategies", in Wilkinson S and Kitzinger C (eds) *Women and Health: feminist perspectives*, Basingstoke, Taylor Francis.

Tones K (1995) "Health education as empowerment", *Health Promotion Today*, London, Health Education Authority.

Tones K and Tilford S (1994) *Health Education: effectiveness, efficiency and* equity, 2nd edn, London, Chapman Hall.

Wellings K, Field J, Johnson AM and Wadsworth J (1994) *Sexual Behaviour in Britain: The National Survey of Sexual Attitudes and Lifestyles*, London, Penguin.

13 Mental health promotion

Deborah Loeb, Wolfgang Markham, Jennie Naidoo and Jane Wills

Key points

- National health strategy.
- Defining mental health promotion.
- Models of mental health promotion.
- Evidence of effectiveness.

Overview

This chapter explores how the designation of mental illness as a national priority has created an opportunity for an increased awareness of mental health promotion. There is no history of agreed target areas, widely accepted approaches or effective indicators in mental health promotion. The chapter looks at the scope for mental health promotion by looking at the targets set in the government strategy and the limitations of focusing on severe mental illness. It goes on to look at the scope for mental health promotion in raising awareness of risk factors and early indicators of mental health problems as well as preventive approaches. How different interpretations of mental health have led to very different approaches to mental health promotion are examined, and an inherent confusion between the concepts of mental health and mental illness is acknowledged. It is argued that mental health needs to be viewed not only at an individual level but also at the level of communities and society, and strategies need to encompass complementary activities at these different levels.

Promoting mental health thus entails more than a focus on mental illness and its indicators such as severe depression and anxiety. Two case studies are presented – an education programme for parents and those who work with children to develop self-awareness and to see parenting in a wider social context; and a programme in schools to enhance well-being and emotional health, which includes activities to reduce stress and aggression and raise children's self-esteem. This chapter argues that health promotion is as much about processes and ways of working as the content and outcome of programmes. That is, an activity may be presented in a way which promotes mental health (e.g. involving participation, empowerment and support) or in a way which militates against mental health (e.g. didactic, guilt-inducing and disempowering). Mental health promotion is therefore relevant to the whole population and can be seen as *a way of working*.

The national health strategy

Mental illness is defined by most people within the framework of a medical model of health which sees the individual in terms of symptoms. These symptoms may vary considerably from the comparatively mild to the very severe which necessitate hospitalization.

Example

Mental health problems in society

Mental health problems occur in approximately 50% of people on social workers' caseloads, whether generic mental health or other specialist. Mental illness accounts for:

- 14.5% of NHS inpatient costs;
- 14% of certified sickness absence (DoH, 1993);
- 26% of men report that they suffer from stress very often or quite often;
- 36% of women report that they suffer from stress very often or quite often;
- 42% of people report that problems at work had caused stress in the last year (HEA, 1990).

Depression is the commonest form of mental ill-health in the community: 6% of men and 12–17% of women suffer from depression, half of them long term. 70% of women and 50% of men will consult their GP about mental health problems at some point (Jacobsen *et al.*, 1991).

D   What particular problems are there in setting and implementing targets for mental health?

The "Health of the Nation" strategy identified mental illness as a national priority, setting targets to reduce the suicide rate and improve the "health and social functioning" of mentally ill people (DoH, 1993). The strategy was widely criticized firstly for its emphasis of pathology and illness rather than health and then for its restricted view on mental illness which ignored the vast majority of undiagnosed mental illness which exists in the community.

The World Health Organization (1993) reports that 90% of those who commit suicide are mentally ill at the time of killing themselves and that depression and alcohol are associated with 80–85% of suicides, hence the choice of two targets to reduce suicide rates as an indicator of a reduction in mental health problems. However, the first target to "improve health and social functioning" suggests that there are objective measures and "serve only to perpetuate untested professional assumptions about what constitutes quality or which achievements rank above which others" (MIND, 1991). In addition, the measurement of outcomes in mental health is conceptually problematic. Interventions may reduce symptoms by, for example, the administration of drugs but possibly at the expense of physical and psychological well-being (Sayce, 1993).

D

> In the light of the following evidence would you target particular groups as at risk from suicide?
>
> ■ Suicide among young men has doubled in the last decade and, after road accidents, is the major cause of death in men under 35 (DoH, 1993).
> ■ Suicide among young Indian women who are first generation immigrants is more than double the national average (Raleigh *et al.*, 1990).
> ■ Unemployed people are twice as likely to commit suicide as those in employment (Moser, 1986).

As we saw in Chapter 5, targeting risk factors and behaviours was the basis for the "Health of the Nation" strategy. The revised strategy due in 1998 is likely to focus on the needs of specific population groups. Whilst there has been particular concern at the rising trend in suicides among young men, the social factors which might explain this trend are largely ignored and suicide is seen as a purely psychological phenomenon requiring interventions to assist the individual. Thus the major focus of action has been on raising awareness of primary care workers to indicators of depression, e.g. GP education and the use of protocols by practice nurses in the assessment and management of depression. Primary and social care are also recommended to keep a database of local support agencies. Reducing stigma among the general public in order to encourage those experiencing depression, stress or anxiety to seek help is also a priority.

The Department of Health (1993) identified the following interventions to reduce suicide:

■ Identifying mental illness and depression in primary and social care settings (66% of people consult their GP in the month before a suicide attempt).
■ Assessment and support for those who have previously attempted suicide (people who have attempted suicide in the past are at particular risk in the year after the attempt).
■ Reducing access to methods of suicide, e.g.:
  changes in exhaust emissions;
  targeting suicide "hot spots" such as bridges;
  labelling paracetamol bottles with toxicity warnings.

Activity

> Consider the following examples of health promotion interventions. What do they have in common?
>
> ***Defeat Depression campaign***
> Organized by the Royal College of General Practice and the Royal College of Physicians, this is intended to improve anticipatory care through raising awareness of GPs in training and information

packages; screening for depression and suicide risk through the use of such tools as the General Health Questionnaire.

Counselling in primary care setting

A health centre which offers counselling, psychotherapy, befriending and complementary therapies has managed to reduce GP psychotropic drug expenditure by one third.

Set in Rural Isolation

A project led by Shropshire Health Promotion Unit to raise awareness of suicide among rural farmers and promote existing support services such as the Samaritans. The number of suicides fell from 40 (1991–92) to 25 (1993–94).

All these initiatives locate depression within the individual suggesting that the emphasis of activity needs to be on its early identification. Not only does this ignore environmental factors in mental health problems but there is also the implication that professional interventions are desired and needed. As Rogers *et al.* (1996:42) point out "despite the common assumption that GPs would be more effective if their psychiatric knowledge were increased and more emotional morbidity identified, from a service user's point of view ordinary relating and practical help may be more important." "Mental health" cannot be seen as the sole province of health services as the contributory risk factors span the work of many other sectors. The action summary for NHS and Social Services managers contained in the key area handbook (DoH, 1993) includes the following guidelines:

- Develop good practice to improve mental health in the NHS and the Local Authority workplace.
- Build alliances for health promotion outside the NHS and Local Authority social services.
- Co-ordinate local strategies with the Health Education Authority.

Defining mental health promotion

The concept of mental health

The concept of mental health is much less well understood than the concept of mental illness and there is no widely accepted definition. There has been a tendency to assume that mental illness and mental health are at opposite ends of a single continuum thereby implying that some people are mentally ill and some mentally healthy. Trent (1991) suggests, however, that mental health and mental illness are more usefully seen as separate concepts – on a dual continuum – which acknowledges that everyone has the capacity for both at any one time.

R

Which of the following definitions of mental health comes closest to your own? Are there any other aspects you would wish to include?

■ Mental health is the emotional resilience which enables us to enjoy life and to survive pain, disappointment and sadness. It is a positive sense of well-being and an underlying belief in our own, and others' dignity and worth (HEA, 1996).
■ Mental health includes the following capacities:
  □ the ability to develop psychologically, emotionally, intellectually and spiritually;
  □ the ability to initiate, develop and sustain mutually satisfying personal relationships;
  □ the ability to become aware of others and to empathize with them;
  □ the ability to use psychological distress as a developmental process, so that it does not hinder or impair further development (NHS Advisory Service, 1995).

What is mental health promotion (MHP)?

"Mental health promotion means different things to different people: for some it means the treatment of mental illness; for others it means preventing the occurrence of mental illness; and for others, it means increasing the ability to overcome frustration, stress, problems, enhancement of resilience and resourcefulness." *Norman Sartorius*, former Director of the Division of Mental Health at the World Health Organization

(Hodgson and Abbasi, 1995:6).

This definition summarizes the central complexity of working in mental health promotion and highlights the range of possible interpretations which are based on different ideological perspectives. It also acknowledges the confusion that surrounds the interchangeable use of the terms mental health and mental illness and the expectations that subsequently follow for working practices and the delivery of mental health programmes.

A regional audit of mental health programmes conducted in NE Thames Region in 1993 highlighted the fact that almost anything can be put under the banner of promoting mental health (NE Thames Regional Health Authority, 1993). Health promoters included exercise classes, adult education, child protection awareness programmes and assertiveness training as examples of mental health promotion programmes. However, it supports the view that mental health underpins all health promotion programmes because it is concerned with fundamental processes. These processes, which in themselves have the potential to promote mental health, are referred to in the WHO Health For All Programme (1985) and include:

- community participation, and
- empowerment.

The following case study has been chosen not only because it is explicitly concerned with promoting mental health in a school context but also because it highlights the role that process plays in determining project outcomes. Seeing a major aspect of mental health promotion as being a way of working has been integral to the development of the project.

Case study

Hackney Well-being Project

The Hackney Well-being in Schools Project is a multi-agency pilot project. The project is funded by East London and City Health Authority (ELCHA) and Hackney Social Services to run for three years. It is an action research project, the results of which will help determine the subsequent development of mental health promotion for young people in Hackney schools.

The aims of the project are:

1. To promote well-being in areas identified by the schools involved.
2. To evaluate and disseminate the project findings.

The Well-being Project was established with high expectations. It is illustrative of the demands such a project makes on workers who need to deliver concrete outcomes. In terms of preventive strategies, schools seem an obvious, and perhaps the only, route into reaching adolescents. Schools, however, have their own considerable schedule of responsibilities, as well as their own philosophies, which will influence their response to these issues.

The Well-being Project team consists of a Community Psychologist and a Health Promotion Adviser with administrative back-up. Funding of £17,000 per annum was made available to release teachers in the chosen pilot schools so that they could work alongside the project workers. There is a steering group made up of representatives of health, social services and education.

A key feature of the project is that it takes a whole-school approach to promoting well-being, recognizing that the ethos, organization and social climate of a school has an important influence on young people's behaviour, attainments, self-esteem and confidence. A central belief is that the way in which people work is as important as the outcomes in promoting well-being. In practice this has meant working with all staff, parents and pupils to achieve longer-term organizational changes. Maximizing on existing strengths and resources within the school to ensure the continuation of a programme of change at the end of the project is consistent with a model of empowerment and also acknowledges the project's time limits.

The project team has used the School Development Planning Framework, a process recommended by the then Department of

Education and Science (1991) for planning and implementing school improvement. This is familiar to schools and identifies priorities supported by action plans which can be carried out, evaluated and developed. In each school the process is:

1. identifying needs and priorities for the project as a whole;
2. producing a project development plan with aims, objectives and long-term success criteria;
3. working on individual action plans for each objective, involving key staff and outside agencies, using the seven stage planning and evaluation cycle proposed by Ewles and Simnett (1995);
4. evaluating and amending project development plans;
5. producing an overall evaluation and exit strategy involving strategies to maintain work in the school.

A project development plan in Horizon School included the following objectives:

- Address the needs of girls.
- Develop anti-bullying approaches.
- Improve the school playground.
- Identify multi-agency support available to the school.
- Facilitate parental involvement.
- Develop Personal and Social Health Education (PSHE) curriculum.
- Involve students in developing a positive image of the school.
- Improve behaviour in the school.

These objectives were chosen following a consultation exercise with pupils, parents, and all staff, both teaching and non-teaching. The challenge for the project was to translate a wide range of personal views into activities which had the potential to impact on mental health and well-being.

Although the pilot schools identified their own issues to address, there is extensive literature which supports the areas identified. The review of Hodgson and Abbasi (1995) identifies studies which reveal that girls often experience more stressors in adolescence than boys and respond very differently. This would suggest that MHP programmes should acknowledge gender differences. The problem of bullying and its impact on mental health is being increasingly recognized. Smith and Sharp (1994:7) state that "continued or severe bullying can contribute to long-term problems as well as immediate unhappiness. Children who are bullied at school risk continuing misery and loss of self-esteem, with possible long-term effects; while those who bully others are learning that they can get their own way by abusing power in their relationships with other people." The approach in this project is to address the mental health of both the victim and the bully and recognize the "stressors" that cause people to become bullies.

For many children what takes place in the playground can have a significant effect on their mental well-being. The social interactions that occur in this setting can be greatly affected by the quality of the environment, the kinds of activities that can take place and the quality of supervision. Improving the playground was selected as a way of encouraging pupils to feel more involved in decision making in the school, thereby raising their self-esteem. Some of the areas of action in relation to the playground objective were to:

- involve children, parents, the local community and staff in developing the playground;
- ensure the playground is safe;
- ensure that each student has something to do at playtime;
- reduce the numbers of fights and incidents of bullying;
- make the playground look nicer and provide a quiet as well as an active area.

Models of mental health promotion

One of the challenges facing those involved in MHP is getting a clear picture of its territory. MacDonald and O'Hara (1996) have adapted the work of Albee and Ryan Finn (1993) to show the positive and negative factors affecting mental health (see Figure 13.1). This model suggests that mental health can be promoted by increasing the elements above the dotted line, and by decreasing the elements below it. It also highlights how health is affected by factors at many different levels.

It could be argued that the aims of mental health promotion programmes, at what ever level they are working, can be unified under the epistemological base of theories which are concerned with the psychological and therefore the internal world of the individual (e.g. Piaget (in Philips, 1981); Rogers, 1961) and those which are concerned with the impact of environmental or broader social issues on the individual and acknowledge the fundamental interconnectedness between the individual and his or her environment (e.g. Erikson, 1963, 1980; Bronfenbrenner, 1979). This view is reinforced by the WHO Ottawa Charter (1986) which explicitly recognizes that the mental health of individuals is influenced by public policy and the environment.

Bronfenbrenner (1979) describes society as an ecological environment consisting of a set of "nested structures" or systems which impact on each other – the micro system focusing on the individual, the meso system involving linkage with other settings in which the individual participates, the exo system concerned with policies that impact on the individual but with which there is no direct contact, e.g. workplace policy on maternity/paternity leave, and the macro

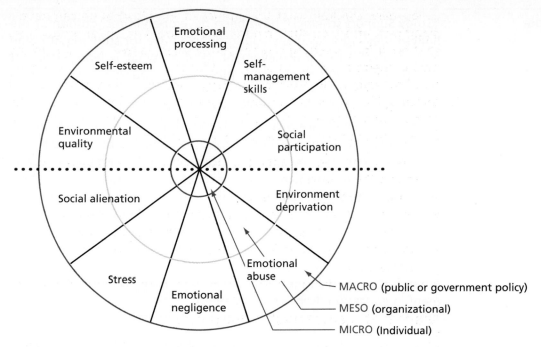

Figure 13.1   *A map of the elements of mental health promotion (adapted from Albee and Ryan Finn, 1993).*

system which represents public or government policy. The key issue is the relationship between these settings. Figure 13.2 shows how a child's ability to learn in school can depend on factors in each system – from the child's personality and ability to parental employment arrangements.

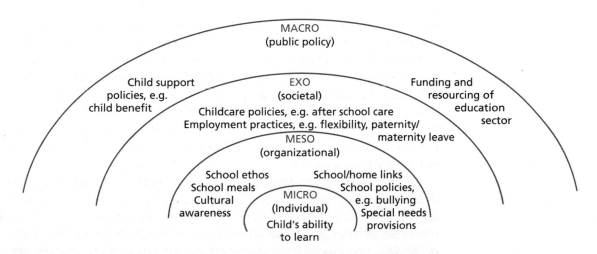

Figure 13.2   *Bronfenbrenner's ecological model of mental health (1979): a child's ability to learn.*

Example

*Applying
Bronfenbrenner's
model*

"Study Support schemes" have been developed in recognition of the limited opportunities many young people have for studying at home and that educational achievement rests on what is learned out of school. Achievement only takes place when young people learn to take responsibility for their own learning. Study Support schemes are usually located in schools or community venues where teachers, students and parents are available to help pupils in their learning. In Tower Hamlets, London, a Study Support scheme has been used by the Education Authority to tackle underachievement. There are currently 27 centres, of which 13 are run by local community groups and which include those for Bangladeshi, African–Caribbean, Chinese/ Vietnamese and Somali young people, and 14 are in mainstream schools. The reported benefits have included increased pupil motivation and self-esteem, improvement in GCSE results and, therefore, increased employment prospects, better preparation for pupils to enter further and higher education, and more community involvement in education (Prince's Trust, 1996).

The view that governments should shoulder a considerable degree of responsibility for the mental health of the individual is supported by the work of Richard Wilkinson (1994, 1996). By drawing on the published material of many authors including himself he was able to demonstrate that social position and relative poverty, i.e. income differences between the rich and poor, are major determinants of health and social problems. Comparisons between developed countries indicate that the most egalitarian societies such as Sweden and Japan enjoy better health as demonstrated by longer average life expectancy and fewer social problems, e.g. lower crime and violence rates than less egalitarian societies such as the UK and USA. Wilkinson argued that in developed countries it is the social rather than the economic implications of relative inequality that has the greatest effect. He concluded that relative inequality directly affects the social cohesion within a society. As a result, egalitarian societies enjoy stronger community life, higher morale, greater social participation and more supportive networks. The psycho-social pathways that are involved in producing greater or lesser social cohesion within a society also impact on the health of all individuals, the privileged as well as the under-privileged. Hence the link between equality and health is, he suggests, largely psycho-social.

The model in Figure 13.3 illustrates the relationship between psychological and social perspectives. It highlights that individuals are continually adapting to stressful events either positively or negatively which occur in a particular context. It also shows that individuals can

Figure 13.3 *Psycho-social perspectives on mental health (Adapted from Hodgson and Abbasi, 1995, with permission).*

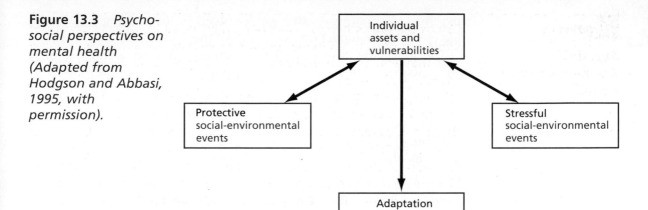

impact on their environment – a fundamental principle of empower-ment. The capacity to do this is influenced by:

- individual assets, e.g. coping skills;
- protective interactions with the environment, e.g. social relationships;
- individual vulnerabilities, e.g. low self-esteem;
- disruptive environments, e.g. parental divorce.

Hodgson and Abbasi (1995) suggest that an important aspect of indi-vidual assets and vulnerabilities is the meaning that an individual gives to a particular stress, e.g. some children respond to starting school very positively – others find it very difficult. These stresses often occur at recognized stages within the developmental life-cycle and are seen as times of "transition" (Erikson, 1959). A role for men-tal health promotion is to help strengthen the ability of individuals to cope with these transition phases, e.g. starting school, adolescence and childbirth, which occur at each developmental stage of life and are potential crisis points.

Some sources of stress – often called "life events", do not however occur at predictable times and often it is the fact that they come at unexpected times which makes them particularly stressful. The meaning that people give to adverse life events can greatly affect a person's health and well-being. For example, Rosengren *et al.* (1993) observed an association between increased mortality and middle-aged men who had recently experienced three adverse life events. This association remained after smoking, self-perceived health, occu-pational status and indices of social support had been taken into account. The life events that seemed to have the greatest effect were serious concern about a family member, being forced to move house, feelings of insecurity at work, serious financial trouble and legal prosecution. As with relative inequality it is likely that the psycho-social pathways that are involved in responding to adverse life events also impact on the health of the individual.

The following case study is an example of a programme which attempts to acknowledge the importance of these experiences in people's lives and how they impact on their decision making processes. Parenting is arguably the most important role many people perform – with the least preparation, education and support. Parenting is not simply a matter of child-rearing. It involves the development of relationships between parents and children, both of whom continue to develop and grow throughout the life cycle. Parenting is also about coping with the diverse pressures in the social and economic environment which can impact on a family.

One of the challenges of becoming a new parent is not only coping with powerful feelings in relation to having a baby but also the likelihood of triggering memories of our own childhood experiences and family relationships. It is increasingly recognized that parents faced with choices about how to bring up their children can benefit from developing an understanding of themselves, their own experiences as children and the values, attitudes, and beliefs of their own families. Without this opportunity the only models that people may have available to them on which to base their parenting style is that used by their own parents – which may not have been completely satisfactory. Negative experiences can get passed on to children in unhelpful ways, albeit unwittingly.

Case study

Background to Parenting

"Background to Parenting" is a course developed in Southern Derbyshire with the aim of bringing an empowerment approach to parenting which promotes non-violence. It evolved out of the expressed needs of parents and those who work with children and parents to understand more about the complex emotions associated with the role of parenting.

Background to Parenting courses work within the framework of the Ottawa Charter and take an ecological approach to parenting, i.e. see people as developing persons living in context with the immediate and wider environment. They encourage and promote a balance between increased and developing personal self-awareness and the need to strengthen community support and responsibility.

Participants are not primarily concerned with running parenting courses or groups, although some do. There is a recognition by participants that many people besides parents have an impact on the lives of children – childcare agencies, nurseries, child protection agencies, schools, women's refuges and the media. Course participants have included people from health visiting, social work, faith communities, community development, parent organizations, education and child protection.

The core elements of Background to Parenting courses are looking at the needs of parents; family types; and parenting styles, understanding developmental stages and times of transition (a life cycle approach described on page 265), the rights of children, tools for parenting, needs assessment and designing a parenting programme. The course encourages participants to develop a working philosophy to support an empowerment approach to parenting issues and a checklist for ensuring that working practices support this philosophy. A checklist for a parenting programme might include the following questions:

- Does the programme question the values base of what is socially acceptable rather than promoting conformity to a particular type of socially acceptable or desirable behaviour?
- Is it culturally aware rather than conforming to a dominant culture?
- Does the programme promote partnership or shared parenting approaches and regard children and parents as developing persons rather than reinforcing roles and stereotypes?
- Does it balance the need for skills with the need to explore the purpose of behaviour and the psychological/social needs of children and parents rather than focusing solely on the development of skills for managing behaviour?
- Does it view parents and children in context within the wider environment and address the need for adequate income, housing and childcare; and equal opportunities?
- Is the programme based on an empowerment model?
- Do the initiatives work towards the development of policies which support parents?
- Is there provision for parents to be involved in the process of policy development?

The Southern Derbyshire Families and Parenting Forum is an initiative whose development has been closely linked to the courses. The forum's aim is to encourage multidisciplinary working and to identify the links between family violence and institutional and other forms of abuse. Its activities involve people from all sectors of the local community. The courses have reflected needs identified within the forum and the forum has been able to promote the existence of the courses and support identified initiatives.

It is in some senses surprising that health promotion activities have not been more closely identified with parenting issues. The scope for promoting health in this potentially fraught area of life is considerable. It is, however, profoundly value-laden and it is therefore essential that programmes are not prescriptive and take place within an empowerment model.

The approach taken in "Background to Parenting" acknowledges that there is a body of theoretical knowledge to which people often do not have access and which can enable them to develop their own views – freeing them from a dependence on their own role models. Course participants become aware that parenting does not take place in isolation from the wider society. Issues of power, hierarchy, gender, cultural diversity, sexuality and inequality need also to be addressed at the societal level. Bronfenbrenner's model on page 263 shows the central interconnectedness between individuals and the meso, exo and macro levels of society. An opportunity to influence the pattern of this interconnectedness is opened up by looking at how policies impact on families.

The health and well-being of an individual (or community) is determined by their ability or inability to develop adaptive coping strategies. Everybody experiences stressors throughout their lives and people cope with these in a variety of ways. However, people who have developed adaptive coping strategies are better able to understand and explain the origins of their stress, feel that they are able to respond effectively, learn from inappropriate or unsuccessful responses and are likely to be able to strike a balance between being reactive and pro-active (Antonovsky, 1987).

The ability to develop these strategies is dependent on life experiences and "generalized resistance resources". Examples of life experiences that promote the development of adaptive coping strategies include consistency and participation in socially-valued decision making. These experiences are affected in turn by work, family structure, gender, ethnicity, culture and opportunity. Examples of generalized resistance resources, sometimes called protective factors, which promote the development of coping strategies include wealth, ego-strength, cultural stability and social support.

A questionnaire was developed by Antonovsky (1987) which enables practitioners to assess a person's "Sense of Coherence" (SOC) or general ability to cope adaptively (see Table 13.1). It can be used to assess the extent to which a person:

1. understands the stresses that they encounter during the course of living (comprehensibility);
2. wishes to address the stresses (meaningfulness);
3. believes they have the resources to meet the challenge of the stresses (manageability).

The SOC construct does not refer to a specific type of coping strategy. Extensive research indicates that the three themes contained within the SOC construct are applicable to all cultures and situations

	Anna (high SOC)	Barbara (low SOC)
Table 13.1 *Antonovsky's Sense of Coherence Construct*	– discusses with family and friends what is happening in her life and identifies work pressures as stressful.	– is so involved in coping with her stressful job that she hasn't identified its stress-inducing features. Blames herself for feeling tired and irritable all the time.
	– is motivated to tackle her stressful job in order to cope with it and avoid "stress leakage" into other areas of her life.	– believes there is nothing she can do to change her job; that this is the way things are and she is lucky to have a job. All she can do is try to cope and get on with it.
	– is confident that she can have an effect on stressful aspects of her work. Recognizes repeating and unhelpful patterns of behaviour. Has in the past made changes to aspects of her life and circumstances (e.g. moved away from her home town).	– is lacking confidence that anything she can do will affect stress levels but hopes that something will turn up in the future.

in the developed world (Antonovksy, 1993). However, due to different life experiences, different groups within a society will have varying average measures of SOC.

Antonovsky (1996) maintained that a person's SOC is stabilized by the end of young adulthood and that thereafter unless a person undergoes major changes in the patterns of life experiences it will only show minor fluctuations. The development of coping strategies in childhood and adolescence is thus of primary importance. Negative feelings towards self and others and problem behaviours can develop in childhood. Hodgson and Abbasi (1995) suggest that working with young people around coping with feelings; developing social skills and good peer relationships as well as positive attitudes to school can all be enhanced between the ages of 6 and 16.

Effective mental health promotion

A difficulty facing practitioners is that there has been comparatively little published evaluation of mental health promotion programmes in the UK as borne out by a literature review conducted by Health Promotion Wales (Hodgson and Abbasi, 1995) and by a forthcoming review from the Health Education Authority even though it is recognized that there is a considerable body of work which might legitimately be seen as mental health promotion taking place.

The effectiveness review by Hodgson and Abbasi (1995) highlighted that most effective interventions in mental health promotion were highly focused or targeted approaches rather than more general mental health programmes. They concluded that there are general protective factors linked to mental health across most developmental stages:

- coping skills;
- good family and social relationships;
- health promoting environments;
- meaningful activities.

They also suggest that there are specific stressors at different developmental stages and that these need to be addressed. They suggested that interventions can be applied to:

- the whole population;
- the population within a developmental stage, e.g. infants; school-age children; adults; older people;
- at-risk or vulnerable groups;
- individuals with a recent mental health or behaviour problem;
- those with a severe mental health or behavioural problem or diagnosed mental illness.

Hodgson and Abbasi (1995) were able to identify more than 40 effective interventions aimed at promoting mental health. Hosman and Veltman (1994) refer to a metastudy (Bosma and Hosman, 1990) on the effectiveness of preventive and mental health promotion interventions aimed at influencing determinants of mental health using international computer searches in several disciplines. They concluded that, in general, child-oriented programmes were more effective than adult-oriented ones. Programmes were particularly successful in:

- improving competence (e.g. social skills, stress management);
- reducing physical risk factors (e.g. prematurity and birth complications);
- improving social health (e.g. job opportunities, school success).

Hosman and Veltman (1994) suggest that given the multicausality of mental health and mental disorders and multiple connections between target groups and their social networks a multicomponent approach would increase the effectiveness of programmes. They conclude that effective mental health promotion interventions:

- aim to influence a combination of several risk or protective factors, e.g. communication and problem-solving skills when preventing marital discord (multifactor);

- involve the social network of the target group such as parents, teachers or family (multisystem);
- include interventions which take place over different times rather than once only (multimoment);
- use a combination of methods, e.g. social support and coping skills (multimethod).

It should be noted that the stringent selection criteria of effectiveness reviews (see Chapter 3) means that only interventions with clear outcome measures are assessed, e.g. preventing separation or relationship satisfaction. As we saw in Chapter 3 the methodologies used in such reviews are not appropriate for evaluating programmes that are based on community participation and empowerment strategies. In these circumstances it may be argued that information regarding process and people's lived experience may be equally important.

Conclusion

This chapter has shown that the mental *health* of individuals needs to be seen as fundamentally connected to the socio-economic, cultural and environmental context in which they are living. Focusing on suicide rates and severe mental illness ignores many of the potential causal factors associated with mental illness as well as mental health. These causal factors are extremely complex and cannot be seen as arising exclusively from biological or psychological conditions. The prevention of mental illness and mental health promotion represent different ideologies, although in practice there are considerable overlaps (Clifford Beers Foundation, 1996). Interventions may, for example, focus on developing communication skills and an increased understanding of emotional needs which is a general skill for positive mental health. If the intervention is targeted at new parents, then it may be effective in *preventing* postnatal depression.

Example

For most women giving birth is a profoundly psychological experience, demanding adjustment to a great many changes in a very short space of time. Antenatal provision concentrates almost exclusively on the physical health of the mother and baby, often ignoring the psychological and emotional needs of parents. Evidence shows that the incidence of postnatal depression can be reduced by allowing women an opportunity to talk over their experience of labour, by preparing mothers and fathers for the physical and emotional support that women will need, and by increasing the degree of social support available to women in the early weeks of motherhood (Holden, 1990).

Figure 13.4   *Promoting mental health – a checklist.*

Empowerment

Does the programme increase opportunities for empowerment through:

		Some key questions
Trust building?	How and to what degree? What are the constraints?	Do participants have access to full information about aims and objectives, anticipated outcomes, their role in the programme?
Cross-cultural working?	How and to what degree? What are the constraints?	How are the needs of different cultural groups reflected and respected in the way the programme is organized? Is there active research into cultural issues in the locality?
Working in partnership?	How and to what degree? What are the constraints?	Is there a possibility for establishing the programme jointly with another group/organization who may reflect the interests of the target/user group? Is the target/user group actively included in this process?
User involvement and participation?	How and to what degree? What are the constraints?	Are programme participants encouraged to give their views on its contents and organization and are those views respected? Are participants satisfied with their level of involvement?
Gaining access to knowledge and information?	How and to what degree? What are the constraints?	Are there opportunities for participants to gain more information and a greater understanding of the programme?
Promoting equity?	How and to what degree? What are the constraints?	Is the principle of equity reflected in the way the programme is organized – is it equally accessible to all; is it located where it is most needed; is the training appropriate for the greatest number of people?

Addressing gender issues?	How and to what degree? What are the constraints?	Do gender issues influence the programme/activity itself and/or its content?
Consciousness-raising?	How? Where?	How are issues presented? What is included, what is excluded and why?
Development of life-skills?	How? Where?	What skills are needed to fully participate in the programme/activity? Is their development being encouraged?
Challenging existing patterns of decision making?	How? Where?	Do programme participants understand how decisions which affect them get made and how to influence them?
Creating supportive networks?	How? Where?	Is there scope to develop a network which might make the programme or activity more immediately effective or long lasting in its effects?
Addressing underlying feelings of powerlessness?	How?	Do all participants feel included or only some of them?
Will the way in which the programme is carried out leave the people, networks, community groups, setting etc. "empowered" as well as achieving the programme objectives?	How?	What long-term positive effects will the programme leave behind it?
Acknowledging that people are the "experts" about their own lives and experiences and is there a recognition of their skills?	How?	What opportunities are there for people to talk about their individual experiences?
Establishing confidentiality where this is appropriate?	How?	How is confidentiality defined by the group?

Mental health promotion is an emerging field of interest for many practitioners but as Tudor points out "In practice, people are either promoting mental health quietly; struggling with what MHP is; or claiming anything remotely to do with mental health and/or mental illness as MHP which only muddies the debates and diminishes the notion" (Tudor, 1996:5). This chapter has shown that there is a role for health promotion in the following:

- Working at a policy level to demonstrate that a key aspect of MHP is that it should be seen as a way of working and that the manner in which institutions such as nurseries, schools, hospitals, training establishments operate can directly impact on mental health, e.g. a healthy workplace policy which examines communication and relationships within the organization and is committed to introducing changes to increase participation and control.
- Involvement in specific targeted initiatives which are based on an empowerment model, e.g. relationships education for school pupils.
- Highlighting the need to develop an understanding of issues associated with psychological and emotional health which should be accessible to individuals at different life stages and in different settings, e.g. pre-retirement courses.

Dodd and Loeb (1994) developed a mental health check list as a tool to support practitioners who wish to promote mental health as part of their work (see Figure 13.4). It is not a blueprint but a guide which can be adapted to suit practitioners' own needs as can be seen in the case study on "Background to Parenting".

 ctivity

The checklist on page 272 provides some criteria to identify whether health promotion programmes empower their participants or target group. Apply these criteria to a health promotion programme with which you are familiar:

- Which criteria does the programme meet?
- Which criteria are not met?
- Can you identify which factors act as barriers to meeting these criteria for promoting mental health?
- Do you agree with all these criteria?
- Are there any other criteria you would add?

Further discussion

- How would you define the difference between mental health promotion and the prevention of mental illness?
- Which approach do you think is most widely adopted and why?

Recommended reading

- Boxer J and McCulloch G (1997) *Mental Health Promotion: Policy, Practice and Partnerships*, London, Baillière Tindall.
  A readable and accessible text which explores definitions of mental health promotion and identifies strategic approaches for practitioners and service users.

- Hodgson R and Abbasi T (1995) *Effective mental health promotion: literature review*, Health Promotion Wales, Technical Report 13.
  A review of recent research providing information on risk and protective factors relating to mental health problems as well as a summary of effective mental health interventions across the life cycle.

- Trent DR and Reed C (eds) *Promotion of mental health*, Vols 1–6 Avebury.
  Each volume is a collection of papers from the annual "Options for Life" European conference on the promotion of mental health which started in 1991.

- Tudor K (1996) *Mental health promotion: paradigms and practice*, London, Routledge.
  A detailed critical analysis of the underlying assumptions, concepts and models of mental health, mental illness and community-based interventions. This book presents a thorough overview of the field but requires serious reading.

References

Albee GW and Ryan Finn KD (1993) "An overview of primary prevention", *Journal of Counselling Psychology*, **72**(2), 115–23.

Antonovsky A (1987) *Unravelling the mystery of health*, San Francisco, Jossey-Bass Inc.

Antonovsky A (1993) "The structure and properties of the sense of coherence scale", *Social Science Medicine*, **36**, 725–33.

Antonovsky A (1996) "The Salutogenic model as a theory to guide health promotion", *Health Promotion International*, **11**, 11–18.

Bosma MWM and Hosman CMH (1990) *Preventie op waarde geschat*, Niijmegen, Beta.

Bronfenbrenner U (1979) *The ecology of human development. Experiments by nature and design*, Cambridge, Massachusetts, Harvard University Press.

Clifford Beers Foundation (1996) *Enhanced mental health promotion and prevention in Europe:*

A Policy Paper, Stafford, Clifford Beers Foundation.

Department of Health (1993) *Key area handbook: Mental illness*, London, HMSO.

Dodd C and Loeb D (1994) "Mental health – a way of working", in Trent DR and Reed C (eds) *Promotion of Mental Health*, Vol. 40, Ashgate, Aldershot.

Erikson E (1959) *Family transitions: Continuity and change over the life cycle*, New York, Guildford Press.

Erikson E (1963) *Childhood and society*, revised edn, New York, W.W. Norton. (Harmondsworth, Penguin 1965.)

Erikson E (1980) *Identity and the life cycle: A re-issue*, New York, W.W. Norton.

Ewles L and Simnett I (1995) *Promoting health: A practical guide*, 3rd edn, London, Scutari Press.

HEA (1990) *Health facts*, London, Health Education Authority.

HEA (1996) *Mental health fact sheet*, London, Health Education Authority.

Hodgson R and Abbasi T (1995) *Effective mental health promotion: literature review*, Health Promotion Wales, Technical Report 13.

Holden J (1990) "Emotional Problems Associated With Childbirth", in Alexander J, Levy V, and Roch S (eds) (1990) *Midwifery practice: Postnatal care*, Basingstoke, Macmillan.

Hosman C and Veltman N (1994) *Prevention in mental health: A review of the effectiveness of health education and health promotion*, Utrecht, International Union for Health Promotion and Education/Dutch Centre for Health Promotion and Education.

Jacobson B, Smith A and Whitehead M (1991) *The nation's health: A strategy for the 1990s*, London, King's Fund.

MacDonald G and O'Hara K (1996) "Ten elements of mental health, its promotion and demotion: Implications for practice", Paper presented at *Options for Life – the Sixth Annual European Conference on the Promotion of Mental Health*, London.

MIND (1991) *Comments on the government's green paper "Health of the Nation"*, London, MIND.

Moser K, Fox A and Jones D (1984) "Unemployment and mortality in the OPCS longitudinal study", *Lancet*, **(ii)**, 1324–9.

North East Thames Regional Health Authority (1993) *Mental health promotion audit*, "Health of the Nation" Focus group on Mental Health, NE Thames RHA.

NHS Advisory Service (1995) *Together we stand: Child and adolescent mental health services*, London, HMSO.

Philips JL (1981) *Piaget's theory: A primer*, San Francisco, W.H. Freeman.

Prince's Trust (1996) *A breakthrough to success study support: A Review*, London, The Prince's Trust.

Raleigh SV, Bulusi L and Balarajan R (1990) "Suicides among immigrants from the Indian subcontinent", *Journal of Psychiatry*, **156**, 46–50.

Rogers CR (1961) *On becoming a person*, London, Constable.

Rogers A and Pilgrim D, with Latham M (1996) *Understanding and promoting mental health*, London, Health Education Authority.

Rosengren A, Orth-Gomer K, Wedel H and Wilhemsen (1993) "Stressful Life Events, Social Support and Mortality in Men Born in 1933", *British Medical Journal*, **307**, 1102–05.

Sayce L (1993) "Improving mental health in Britain: a commentary on the 'Health of the Nation'", *Journal of Mental Health*, **2**, 305–313.

Smith PK and Sharp S (1994) *School Bullying: Insights and perspectives*, London, Routledge.

Trent D (ed.) (1991) *Promotion of mental health*, Vol 1, Aldershot, Avebury.

Tudor K (1996) *Mental health promotion: Paradigms and practice*, London, Routledge.

WHO (1993) *Guidelines for primary prevention of mental neurological and psychosocial disorders*, No 4, Geneva, World Health Organization.

Wilkinson R G (1994) *Unfair shares: The effects of widening income differentials on the welfare of the young Barnardos*, Ilford, Essex, Barnardos.

Wilkinson R G (1996) *Unhealthy societies: The afflictions of inequality*, London, Routledge.

Index

Numbers in *italic* refer to illustrations; numbers in **bold** refer to tables